The Journey
to Radiant Health

Prema Key

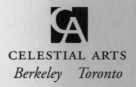

CELESTIAL ARTS
Berkeley   Toronto

Celestial Arts
P.O. Box 7123
Berkeley, California 94707
www.tenspeed.com

Distributed in Australia by Simon & Schuster Australia, in Canada by Ten Speed Press Canada, in New Zealand by Southern Publishers Group, in South Africa by Real Books, and in the United Kingdom and Europe by Airlift Book Company.

LIBRARY OF CONGRESS CATALOGING-IN-PUBLICATION DATA

Key, Prema Scott.
    The journey to radiant health / Prema Scott Key. — 1st ed.
        p.   cm.
    Includes bibliographical references.
    ISBN 1-58761-175-9 (pbk.)
    1. Health—Religious aspects.   I. Title.
BL65.M4K39   2003
299'.93—dc22   200   3024151

Printed in Canada

FIRST PRINTING, 2003

1 2 3 4 5 6 7 8 9 10 — 07 06 05 04 03

This book is humbly placed
before the Enlightened Beings
that inspired it;
Avatar Sathya Sai Baba,
Mahavatar Babaji
and the Pleadians.

May its contents provide loving assistance
to all Souls on the path to greater awareness.

ABOUT THE AUTHOR

Prema Scott Key has worked in the fields of holistic health and spiritual counseling since 1990. His own healing journey led him to develop a holistic, integrative counseling model that addresses all three bodies—emotional, mental and physical—and promotes core-level healing. Prema also offers clients homework assignments that emphasize action as a pathway to accelerated spiritual growth.

Prema's certifications include Acupressure Technician with a specialization in Emotional Balancing, Yoga instructor, Massage Therapist, and Color Therapy Practitioner. He has also studied with Michael Harner, author of *The Way of the Shaman*, and Ron Teeguarden, Tonic Herbalist and author of *Radiant Health*.

Prema leads group retreats, seminars and workshops that offer simple spiritual principles and practices to elevate awareness, and facilitate physical, mental and emotional health and healing. Prema has hosted *Love Is the Action*, a cable television show dedicated to healing dis-ease and raising conscious awareness.

PREFACE

The Journey to Radiant Health is a manual for living in the new millennium. The information contained in this book can help you recognize and break free of limitations, and create a positive direction for your life.

You will come to understand your true nature and realize your potential, not by concepts, but by actions. With more than thirty exercises and practices, you will find what you need to live from your heart, and bring your dreams to reality. The seven steps on *The Journey to Radiant Health* will help you build and maintain a level of conscious awareness that will open your heart and mind, and bring you into alignment with your own Divinity.

Also included are two dynamic models that will assist you in your quest to experience Radiant Health.

Conscious breathing, the first model, and the foundation of Radiant Health, will expand your awareness and keep you focused, alert and present in the here and now. In the section on Conscious Breathing, you will also learn about its profound health-producing and life-altering effects.

The second model, The Sacred Trinity of Radiant Health, is an exciting paradigm for healing. While modern science uses dissection to study and treat dis-ease, The Sacred Trinity of Radiant Health uses the Spiritual principle of integration to reunite the three bodies—emotional, mental and physical. Integrate the three bodies and you establish a deeper connection with your true nature, Spirit.

Integration also facilitates core-level healing.

The universal stability found in the triangle of The Sacred Trinity of Radiant Health will enable you to integrate and express the Spiritual ideal found in the center of each body. By asserting the Sacred Trinity's, and *The Journey to Radiant Health's* core message *"Love is the highest Truth one can put into Action,"* you will experience wholeness.

The Sacred Trinity of Radiant Health also explores the intrinsic energetic qualities associated with the three bodies: feminine, masculine and Divine Child. It will help you understand the nature of the three bodies, and show you how to integrate your masculine and feminine energies. Integration will enable you to bring the Divine Child into existence—the balanced, harmonious and joy-filled Spirit-self that lives fully in the moment without fear.

The three sections that follow The Sacred Trinity of Radiant Health explore the individual components of the three bodies. Each section provides detailed information on how to recognize and avoid the onset of dis-ease and build the supreme state of emotional, mental and physical health that enables you to experience Radiant Health.

Finally, the Appendix contains Meridian and Chakra system charts (the subtle energy structures related to the physical body) along with detailed explanations of how to use them to release blockages of energy and return to Radiant Health.

There is no time like the present to make the decisions that will enable you to realize your true nature and experience the greatest joy.

ACKNOWLEDGMENTS

Thank you God for all the love, support and lessons you have provided in the creation of this book.

Heart-felt thanks to my late wife, Toni Marie Key, for your unending love, support, editing and for naming the book.

Sharon Bear, Ph.D., and Megan Keefe: editing.

Christine Collings, M.A., editing and illustrator of the Meridian charts and Chakra System charts.

David Sand: cover art.

Dottie Albertine: chart designs.

Brian Treffeisen: chart revision and conscious breathing illustration.

Susan Aldrich and Leon Proknik: initial evaluations.

MaryKay Adams: initial editing.

Ayn Cates, Ph.D.; spiritual support, friendship and editing.

Brent Maddock, Birgit and Marie Funch, Dan Ganglehoff, Frankie Coleman, Kathi Close, Ellen Francisco, Larry Gilmour, comments and edits.

Marie Litster: fine-tuning the Meridian and Chakra illustrations.

So many people contributed to this project, and if your name has been omitted please know that it was not intentional.

TABLE OF CONTENTS

SECTION FIVE

INTRODUCTION

We have entered a period of time unlike any in recorded history. The challenges we face on a personal and worldwide scale are enormous. Corruption, greed, rampant violence, global warming, species extinction, deforestation, toxic and nuclear waste, destruction of the environment, shrinking food supplies, air and water pollution and overpopulation are just a few.

But there is hope. . . . and help.

At least five different cultures handed down prophecies that addresses this time period. When studied carefully, they clearly and specifically forecast the challenges we currently face. They also reveal that, individually and collectively, our future will be determined by the choices we make, right now!

Advances made in scientific fields, such as quantum physics, have provided us with a body of information that now support what Spiritual disciplines have proclaimed for millennia.

You are Spirit.

Science now confirms that you are composed of light. Light is Spirit, and Spirit is consciousness. Today, planet Earth is being bathed with more Light than has been seen in thousands of years. Simply stated, the increase in Light translates to amplified information which can be used to broaden your awareness. Tap into the Light and you can make conscious, healthy decisions to experience and express love and truth, and create a clear and satisfying direction for your life.

SECTION ONE

. . . love produces a very high frequency
while the frequency of fear is substantially lower.

Starting the Journey

*The Journey of a Thousand Miles
starts with the First Step.*
—*Chang Tzu*

If you feel challenged, overwhelmed or things have been downright difficult, take heart in the following information. At the present time there is a subtle and yet major energy shift taking place on Earth. The shift is unlike anything that has come before it, and its ability to help effect change in your life is unprecedented. Specifically, its energy can be used to dispel fear from your mind, and draw love into your heart.

As is the case with every human being, free will gives you the choice of whether to take advantage of this opportunity. Choose to use this energy and you will experience a complete transformation of conscious awareness, one that will empower you to achieve Radiant Health.

The shift is a movement away from Darkness.

The energy that can help you effect change is Light.

The Effects of More Light

Light is information.

Information is the power behind the understanding and awareness that facilitates healing and Radiant Health. On *The Journey to Radiant Health*, Light will be used to ascertain where we have been, where we are and where we are going.

With each passing day, Earth is being exposed to more Light.

The available Light can expand your conscious awareness, illuminating the fundamental truth about who you are in reality, a truth which has long been hidden from you by the Darkness.

The Common Names of Light

Words or ideas used to describe Light include: Goddess or God, Great Spirit, the Tao, Allah, Yahweh or the Creator, inner guidance, conscious awareness, information, energy, love, wisdom, truth or Agape. While the words can change, what does not is its effect. Anything exposed to Light has an opportunity to grow. Right now, you have an unprecedented opportunity to eliminate the Darkness and transform the constrictive, unhealthy, dis-eased energies that it produces—ignorance and fear—into expansive, healthy and harmonic energies including peace, love and greater conscious awareness.

The Shift from Darkness to Light

To better understand the shift from Darkness to Light, consider this: everything in the visible universe is subject to dualistic cycles. Our sun's cyclical and orbital pattern draws it near the hub of our galaxy, and then away from it. This hub is known as the *Grand Center.*

Our sun's orbital pattern is divided into two equal cycles: ascending and descending. Our sun and solar system move towards the Grand Center during the ascending cycle and away from it during the descending cycle.

Each ascending and descending cycle takes approximately 12,000 years to complete. The closer the sun is to the Grand Center, the more Light is available; the further away from the Grand Center, the less. According to the Vedas—ancient books of knowledge—each cycle is further divided into four ages or Yugas. In order from descending to ascending the four are: The Kali Yuga/Iron/Material Age is 1,200 years in duration, and marks the first stage of the development of mental virtue. During this age the human intellect cannot comprehend the fine matters of creation or anything beyond the gross material of the external world.

The Dwapara Yuga/Copper/Atomic Age is 2,400 years in duration and is the age in which the human intellect is able to comprehend the fine matters or electricities and their attributes which are the creating principles of the external world. The Treta Yuga/Bronze/Mental Age is 3,600 years in duration, and in this age the human intellect attains the capacity to comprehend the Divine magnetism, which is the source of all electrical forces on which creation depends for its existence.

The Satya Yuga/Golden/Spiritual Age is 4,800 years in duration. During the Satya Yuga the mental virtue is completely and fully developed and the human intellect can comprehend everything including God, the Spirit beyond the visible world.

The completion of our sun's descending cycle occurred in the year 399 A.D., marking its furthest orbital point away from the Grand Center, and our darkest year—in terms of the availability of Light needed to achieve Spiritual illumination. Our sun's ascending cycle and its return to the Grand Center began immediately thereafter in the year 400 A.D.[1]

But, the dark ages were not over.

The descending Kali Yuga was followed immediately by the ascending Kali Yuga. In all, the descending and ascending Kali Yugas lasted a total of 2,400 years—from 801 B.C. to 1599 A.D.

The Effects of Darkness

During the Kali Yugas, the reduced amount of available Light causes the collective consciousness of humanity to fall under the spell of Darkness, and rulers to come to power by the use of force and by propagating fear.

The Darkness causes humanity to forget its true nature.

Humanity's true nature is that of Light.

Recorded history validates that during the Kali Yugas, humanity was besieged by ignorance. In the midst of the Darkness, the guiding principles and qualities of love were forgotten. War, pestilence and suffering were commonplace. Humanity's ability to live in peace and harmony were lost. To this day, humanity struggles to embrace the Light and exhibit its loving qualities such as peace, non-violence, truth and right conduct.

In a sense, the Darkness caused a power outage, triggering amnesia in the collective conscious. As humanity forgot its own Spiritual nature, balance and harmony were lost. The result is described as the Cartesian split: the division between heart and mind, and the separation of humanity from its own Divinity. What followed was the birth of hierarchical structures and patriarchal religions that depict humanity as being separate from God and women as subservient to men.

Over the course of thousands of years, the Darkness inherent in these and other man-made myths have become interwoven in the psychic fabric of the collective consciousness of humanity. The effects of the Darkness are still evident in modern society in the hierarchical structures and patriarchal religions that are the hallmarks of competitive and authoritarian dominator cultures.

But the truth cannot be changed.

You are Spirit.

Your true nature is Divinity encased in human form and you are made of Light.

You chose to incarnate on Earth to advance Spiritually by overcoming the Darkness. Remember this truth and you will reclaim the Light of your own Divine nature and help extricate the Darkness from the collective consciousness.

The Return to Light

The dark ages continued for the next 1,200 years as our solar system moved through the ascending Kali Yuga. More importantly, however, is that it began moving back towards the Grand Center. Slowly, as more Light became available, the intellectual capacity of humanity began to expand. In 1600 A.D., the electrical age or "Dwapara Yuga" was ushered in and during its entry phase, the presence of electricity was discovered in all material substances. In 1720 A.D., Stephen Gray detected electrical activity in the human body and humanity began to make rapid progress in all scientific fields.

Using Light to Help You Achieve Radiant Health

The Light enables you to reclaim your Divine nature and reawaken to Spirit, because Light exposes and eradicates Darkness. Light is your ally, beckoning you to invite her into your heart. Permit her to and she will help you vanquish the Darkness. Accepting her invitation might seem simple, but in practice it can be quite a challenge. After all, the Darkness that can infringe on your mind is not always your own.

The Seeds of Darkness and Fear

The seeds of Darkness and fear were planted in the collective human consciousness as the sun began to move away from the Grand Center, its source of Light. As the seeds took root, they grew to envelop the consciousness of all humanity. Since its inception, the toxic dis-eases of ignorance and fear produced by Darkness have been passed from generation to generation, building momentum and growing stronger. The memory of Darkness and fear is now so deeply imprinted in our DNA that the feelings they produce are familiar and considered ordinary, even though they are completely unhealthy. The problem is that as familiarity creates a sense of comfort, it also creates a resistance to change. To identify and eradicate the resistance a practice is needed to produce awareness. The seven steps to Radiant Health (page 10) will assist you in that endeavor.

To unravel and eradicate the imprints of Darkness you must engage in a process to awaken. You will have to make a decision to achieve a higher level of conscious awareness, one that will enable you to recognize your true nature and unearth and discard all behaviors, perceptions, attitudes and patterns rooted in Darkness and fear.

The Light is ready to help you.

She offers you the opportunity to realize the dream of Radiant Health. A dream so powerful, so dynamic, and yet, until this point in time, so shrouded by Darkness that few have been able to even imagine it, let alone achieve it. Still, the legacy left by those that sought and achieved Radiant Health is one of inspiration and unlimited possibility.

The Journey to Radiant Health

Up until now, the journey to actualize the dream of Radiant Health could only be likened to embarking on a monumental pilgrimage. Although there are no mountains to climb or seas to cross, it spans the greatest distance one can imagine: the distance between the mind and the heart. It is the heart that will liberate you from the bondage of the mind-based ego, which exists in Darkness. Follow the heart and it will lead you to the path of love.

The path of love is the only path that leads to Radiant Health.

For thousands of years Chinese medicine has defined Radiant Health as "health beyond danger." However, this period of greater and sustained Light elevates the term to new heights, transforming its meaning.

Radiant Health is the supreme state of health and well-being that is produced by living in the heart of love, at one with Spirit.

In essence, the journey has nothing to do with searching for something that exists outside you, but rather it is an inner journey. It is a journey to achieve the balance produced by integrating the emotional, mental and physical bodies. Integration produces balance, the ability to give and receive love. And not just ordinary love but the highest form of love, Agape. Agape is defined as *spontaneous self-giving love expressed freely without calculation of cost or gain to the giver or merit on the part of the receiver*. As you disengage from the mind's fear and chatter and tune into the voice of the heart, the dream of Radiant Health will become a reality.

Everything you need to achieve Radiant Health exists within you. The Light, and its angels and guides, are ready to assist your process of awakening. They await your invitation. The Light can help you resolve the split between mind and body, and other such Cartesian conflicts and struggles that keep you from realizing that you are whole.

The Light is here to remind you of your Divine nature. Its energy sanctions the marriage between the heart and mind. Using it to form an alliance between the two will help you balance your masculine and feminine energy. Integration will enable you to identify and shatter the belief systems, attitudes and perceptions that make you feel unworthy of God's love.

The Process of Awakening

Awakening into full conscious awareness is essential on your journey to Radiant Health. If you do not wake up, you will spend your life in Darkness, wandering around in the sleep-induced state of Maya, never knowing the Light of your Spirit, and unable to achieve Radiant Health.

Maya is a powerful cosmic force capable of creating the illusion that the phenomenal world is real. Under its spell, Maya causes you to believe that you are separate from God and nature, and are different from other human beings. Maya leads you to believe that you have no power to change and its blinding force also will make you swear that the duality found in the ephemeral world is based in truth.

To dispel the power of Maya and experience Radiant Health, you must undergo a fundamental shift in your state of conscious awareness. A wise Hindu adage states:

It would be very good if we would wake up before we die.

Until now, the only episodes capable of causing such a dramatic shift in conscious awareness were mystical, Spiritual, drug-induced or traumatic. Cloaked in a veil of mystery, these are the kinds of events that have traditionally catalyzed the process of awakening. They open the door to higher conscious awareness and spontaneously rouse individuals from their waking slumber.

After the door has been opened, it cannot be closed.

Opening the Door to Conscious Awareness

The need for you to wait or hope for an event of this magnitude is over. With each new day the Light is changing the playing field. You can now initiate the process of awakening and shift your state of conscious awareness. You or someone you know might have already had this experience. The process of awakening will pay off in greater conscious awareness and emotional, mental and physical health and well-being.

For thousands of years superior health-producing techniques, formulas and systems have existed to treat emotional, mental or physical dis-ease. For the most part, however, they have remained separate from one another. On *The Journey to Radiant Health*, you will work with a number of the most powerful health-producing paradigms. As you put them into practice, they will make an extraordinary difference in your life.

The Seven Steps to Radiant Health

You can achieve Radiant Health by putting the following seven steps into action. Each step increases conscious awareness, bringing you closer to self-realization and the experience of Agape. Steps one and two establish the groundwork for *The Journey to Radiant Health*. The five subsequent steps support step two—putting Love into Action.

Whether you are a beginner on the path to conscious awareness or have already been awakened, the seven steps to Radiant Health will take you to the next level on your journey. Below is a brief overview of the steps.

Step 1. Conscious Breathing.

Conscious breathing is introduced in Section Two and is your foundation on *The Journey to Radiant Health*. Conscious breathing can jump-start the conscious awakening process, expanding your awareness and strengthening your ability to detect the subtle vibrations of energy that exist in all things. Conscious breathing promotes emotional stability, mental clarity and physical health, and facilitates integration of these three aspects. Integration is key to balance—a cornerstone to Radiant Health.

Step 2. Put Love into Action.

"Love is the highest Truth that one can put into Action" is the centerpiece of The Sacred Trinity of Radiant Health, a dynamic model presented in Section Three that consists of the three bodies—emotional, mental and physical—and their basic spiritual qualities: Love, Truth and Action. The application of this Spiritual axiom in your day to day life will enable you to achieve Radiant Health.

Set an intention to put Love into action and the effects are immediate and profound. Love carries and transmits a frequency that enables you to identify and consciously change the words, thoughts, feelings and deeds that arise from fear. It is one of the most challenging tasks that can be undertaken, but the rewards make it well worth the effort.

Steps one and two, when used consistently and in conjunction with one another, raise your frequency, promote greater self-awareness and Spiritual growth, facilitate emotional, mental and physical healing and empower you to recognize and dispel fear. The next five steps support your ability to put Love into action by bringing you into harmony with your Spirit.

Step 3. Pray and Meditate Every Day.

Prayer and meditation, also introduced in Section Three, enable you to establish and maintain sacred communion with the Divine. Prayer is used to ask for guidance and meditation is used to receive it. The two practices keep the heart and mind open, and keep you emotionally centered during times of change, difficulty or crisis. Used daily and in conjunction with one another, prayer and meditation strengthen your focus and conscious awareness, keeping it attuned to the Divine and open to the power of Love.

Step 4. Develop a Relationship with Your Spirit Child.

Soul Loss, the Spiritual origin of dis-ease, leads to a variety of emotional and mental disorders and physical ailments. Soul Loss occurs when a traumatic experience causes part of the soul to split off, becoming fragmented. Your Spirit Child, unveiled in Section Four, can help you identify prior traumas that have resulted in Soul Loss. The Spirit Child is a gatekeeper that can help you access the Spirit world and retrieve the fragments. The retrieval of the fragmented parts of the soul facilitates core-level healing and empowers holistic health. The healing produced by this step restores balance, opens the door to the heart and leads to emotional maturity.

Step 5. Be Honest and Truthful in All your Affairs.

This step brings you face to face with the producer of Darkness, the ego. The heart is the abode of Love and Spirit, and contains the answer to any question. When the primary focus for your actions becomes Love, your conscience will not rest and it will become easy to distinguish ego actions (Darkness) from Love actions (Light). From the Light of truth, miraculous healing and personal transformation can take place.

Step 6. Find and Pursue Your Life's Purpose.

The primary reason for your incarnation on Earth is to fulfill your life purpose. In Section Six you will find an exercise that enables you to uncover your life purpose. When you find and pursue your life purpose you will experience lasting peace, joy and fulfillment.

Step 7. Serve Others.

On *The Journey to Radiant Health* the pursuit of your life purpose is key to your Spiritual evolution and long-term fulfillment. Your life purpose, when put into action, will cause you to serve others naturally. Serving others as often as you can will enable you to minimize suffering and maximize joy.

The seven steps to Radiant Health, and the exercises that support them, will be explored in great detail in following chapters.

2

The World's Journey to Radiant Health

Even though our solar system began its orbital journey towards the Light some 1,600 years ago and is 400 years removed from the ascending Kali Yuga, the Darkness continues to interfere with the collective awakening of humanity. Eventually the Light will propel humanity to its collective awakening and the world to Radiant Health; however, at present the Darkness still has enough energy to prohibit humanity from experiencing a collective awakening.

But all that is about to change.

Long ago a number of tribes and peoples were given clear and detailed messages that spoke of a time in the future when a dramatic shift would transform humanity. Each prophecy states that the shift will end the age of Darkness and move the world into an era of Light. Each also proclaims that harbingers will signal the shift's imminent arrival.

The harbingers have come.

The time to prepare is now.

Prophecy and World Radiant Health

The prophecies that will be reviewed here have been chosen from five distinct tribes or cultures and all adhere to the following criteria: each of the prophecies has either been written or passed on by oral tradition. Each contains the specific local or global events that will indicate the shift is underway. A number of events have already taken place, while others loom over the horizon. The ancient prophecies, along with modern prophets like Edgar Cayce and Nostradamus, indicate that the shift will start somewhere near the end of the millennium and continue into the new millennium. A common theme among the prophecies is that sometime between now and the date December 21, 2012 A.D., humanity will witness the close of one world cycle and the opening of another. The prophecies also assert that when the New Age is ushered in, reality as it has been known, both on a personal and world-wide scale, will be changed forever.

Jewish Prophecy

In the Old Testament of the Holy Bible, Jewish prophets state that three specific events must take place before the new era of peace and harmony on Earth will begin:

1. The Jewish people must be brought back to their homeland (Ezekial 37:11 and 38:8, Matthew 24:32). This historic event took place on May 14, 1948, with the birth of Israel as a nation and the call, by Prime Minister Ben-Gurion, for all Jews to return to their homeland.

2. The Jews must be in possession of the ancient city of Jerusalem (Zechariah 12:11-14 and Matthew 24:15). This prophecy was fulfilled on the third day of the Six-Day War in June 1967, when the ancient city of Jerusalem was taken by the Israelis.

3. The ancient Jewish temple must be rebuilt on its original site, Mount Moriah (Matthew 24:15). At the time of this writing, the Dome of the Rock, the second holiest shrine of the Moslem faith, sits squarely in the middle of the ancient temple site. No one knows how or when the temple will be rebuilt, but prophecy clearly states that the new era of world peace and harmony will not begin before this event takes place. Prophecy also states that the new era will commence within one generation of Israel becoming a nation (Matthew 24:34). This point has stirred debate because during biblical times a generation generally consisted of approximately 40 years. Nonetheless, the fact remains,

according to prophecy, that the three events must take place before the dawn of the new era is witnessed.[1]

A vast number of prophetic messages, including an epic battle between good and evil—Armageddon—are also found in the Book of Revelation. Its messages make reference to this event and others that will be the precursors to the coming age. However, because the messages are in cryptic and symbolic form, no attempt will be made to decode them here.

Hopi Prophecy

Prophecies given to the Hopi nation around 1100 A.D. by Maasaw, the Guardian of the Earth, clearly define the historical close of what the Hopi call the Fourth World Cycle.[2] Many of Maasaw's prophecies have already come to pass and others are now being fulfilled. However, the following nine are said to be the most important. The events have occurred in order and, as with the Jewish prophecies, only one event remains to be fulfilled.

1. White-skinned men will come, take land that is not theirs and strike their enemies with thunder—Guns.

2. The Hopi lands will see the coming of spinning wheels filled with voices—Covered wagons.

3. A strange beast like a buffalo, but with great long horns, will overrun the land in large numbers—Longhorn cattle.

4. Snakes of iron will cross the land—Railroad tracks.

5. A giant spider's web will crisscross the land—Power and telephone lines.

6. Rivers of stone that make pictures in the sun will crisscross the land—Concrete roads and their mirage-producing effects.

7. The sea will turn black, and many living things will die because of it—Oil spills.

8. Many youth, who wear their hair long like the Hopi, will come and join the tribal nations to learn our ways and wisdom—Hippies.

9. A dwelling-place in the heavens, above the Earth, shall fall with a great crash. It will appear as a blue star. This is the final prophecy and is yet to be fulfilled. Could this "dwelling place" possibly be the Space Station?

Other Hopi prophecies that indicate the cycle's closing and that are being fulfilled today include:

1. Children will be out of control and will no longer obey their leaders.—Children are murdering other children and adults with alarming frequency. In the last four years 17,822 children age nineteen and under were killed by guns. Suicide among the age group from fifteen to nineteen doubled between 1970 and 1990. Suicide and homicide currently account for one third of all deaths among teens.[3]

2. Hopi children and even adults will forget their language. The majority of Hopi children do not speak their native tongue.

3. There will be changes in the attitudes and behaviors of the world's people, including increased immorality and materialism as the competitive war of greed flourishes. The world has grown increasingly more materialistic and greedy as nations compete for resources and corporations compete for power.

4. The time will come when we will experience late springs and early frosts; this will be the sign of the returning Ice Age. Each winter has extended further into spring than the previous winter, and early spring frosts have consistently wiped out crops. The earth-warming greenhouse effect plays a big part because of the increasing rise in content of atmospheric carbon dioxide gas. The effect is a changing climate worldwide, droughts, high winds and storms resulting increased erosion and an increase in volcanic activity which results in an increase

in ice at the Earth's poles. Depletion of soil minerals will cause forest and agricultural plants to die. A warming atmosphere causes more evaporation of water from the ocean which means more rain, snow or sleet. The conversion of more water from vapor to precipitation also releases more energy into the atmosphere making storms more powerful . . . a warming climate is expected to produce hotter heat waves and more severe droughts.

The fact that these prophecies were received by the North American Hopi tribe in 1100 A.D., and are being fulfilled in direct correlation with biblical prophecy is stunningly remarkable. Finally, another prophecy proclaims, "The Great day of Purification has been described as a Mystery Egg which will culminate either in total rebirth or total annihilation. At this time's end, there will be a new dawn of time when the world will bloom into peacefulness." This also aligns with Jewish prophecy to proclaim that a new era of harmony will reign after the shift.[4]

Lakota Prophecy

Lakota legend says that before leaving the sacred lodge, White Buffalo Woman passed the sacred pipe to the elders and declared, "I will always return at the end of the four ages." The Native American belief in the four ages parallels the Hindu belief in the four Yugas—ages. A Lakota prophecy, adhered to by many Native American tribes of the northern plains, proclaims, "When a true white buffalo is born, a time of cleansing and healing of the Earth will commence." At that time White Buffalo Woman will return to the Earth to unify the nations of the four colors—black, red, yellow and white—in peace and joy. The prophecy also declares, "To signify the pending unification, during the buffalo's maturing process its coat will mutate, turning each of the colors of the four root races."[5] The transmutation of the white buffalo's coats will signify the pending unification of the root races. Lakota prophecy also asserts that the birth will occur in the seventh generation after the red man has lost his lands.

The seventh generation has arrived.

The White Buffalo is here.

While the odds of the birth of a true white buffalo are one in tens of millions, on August 20, 1994, on Dave Heider's farm in Janesville, Wisconsin, a true white female buffalo calf was born—a true white buffalo is signified by brown eyes rather than the pink eyes of an albino.

Dave's father in-law, Jerry, says that at 5 AM on the morning of August 20, Dave walked outside to start his day and was surprised to see three Native Americans sitting in a car outside his front door. Dave asked them what they were doing there.

"We came to see your white buffalo," they said.

"I don't have a white buffalo," Dave said.

The Native Americans were certain that a white buffalo had been born on the farm and asked Dave to please look in his pen. Skeptical about their claim, Dave begrudgingly walked to the pen in which he kept twelve buffalo. Sure enough there was a thirteenth. Shocked, Dave asked where they were from and how they knew about the buffalo. "We drove from South Dakota," they said. "She came to us in a dream and led us right here to your front door." Stunned and amazed Dave fittingly named her Miracle.

The Native Americans then asked Dave for permission to bring a few of their elders to perform a three day ceremony in honor of the buffalo. Dave agreed and three days later 150 elders arrived. Dave cleared space on his farm to accommodate them. On the fourth day, however, Dave got the jolt of his life; 1,500 Native American elders and chiefs arrived.

From all over the country they came and when Dave asked them how they knew to come here, each said that a dream had led them to this spot. Native American tribal leaders had converged on the farmer's land before the media reported the news of her birth. They came from far and wide, drawn by a sacred vision and divine guidance. They came to acknowledge and honor the sacred white buffalo as the symbolic fulfillment of ancient prophecy and the harbinger of the coming change. The Native Americans' pilgrimage to honor the white buffalo was so profuse that the Cable Network News (CNN) and Associated Press headlined the story. In accordance with prophecy, as Miracle grew and matured, the color of her coat did indeed change four times. Her coat, white at birth, changed color every six months; it first turned black, then yellow and then red. Her coat is now a natural brown and she still lives on the Heider Farm. Dignitaries including the Dalai Lama—Spiritual leader of Tibet—as well as common folks from all over the world have come to pay their respects and honor the birth of the white buffalo, and the fulfillment of the ancient prophecy of White Buffalo Woman.[6]

The birth of Miracle the 13th buffalo, the initial appearance of three Native Americans who were led by a vision, and then others who came to pay their respects, bears an uncanny and remarkable resemblance to the story of the three wise men and others who came to honor the birth of Jesus of Nazareth.

Mayan Prophecy

The origins of the Mayan people remain a scientific enigma, as does the nature of Mayan culture, how it started and why it declined so abruptly. The prophetic Mayan calendar, however, is still hailed as the most mathematically accurate calendar in the world. To date, the efforts of science have not been able to unlock the secret of how the Mayans were able to create a time-keeping system so precise and exact in its measurements. So precise, in fact, that its calculations remain unequaled and unparalleled, even by today's modern exacting standards and scientific methods of time-keeping.

Many who have studied the Mayan, including Jose Arguelles, author of *The Mayan Factor*, believe the Mayan were an extremely advanced culture. The Mayan deftly blended science and Spirituality to attain a level of knowledge that far exceeds that of any modern culture. Believed by some to be a product of this harmonic blending, the prophetic Mayan calendar is so exact that it gives the date, December 21, 2012 A.D.[7], that the Mayans claim will be the close of the fifth world cycle. In accord with the other prophecies discussed, the possibility of Armageddon or Apocalypse also exists.

The Harmonic Convergence

According to the prophetic Mayan calendar, an event that held powerful implications for widespread change was slated to take place on August 16, 1987. According to Mayan prophecy, if 144,000 people could be brought together in meditation at dawn on August 16, the world would be renewed and humanity would enter a "New Age."

The event was called the Harmonic Convergence.

Arguelles, inspired by the possibility of its fulfillment and actualization, traveled around the world to share the prophetic message. He encouraged people everywhere to gather at sacred sites to participate in meditation ceremonies designed to activate the energies of the Harmonic Convergence. Estimates put the participants of the world-wide event at more than one million people for the prescribed day.

According to Mayan prophecy, the Harmonic Convergence marked the beginning of materialism's climax which was slated to occur from 1987 to 1992. During this time period a decision was to be made to either return to the harmonic rhythm of nature or bring on a biospheric collapse. By turning away from the culture of materialism and the manmade, twelve month Gregorian calendar, and returning to living in harmony with nature, which includes observing nature's 13 harmonic cycles of new moons per calendar year, the New Age can be fulfilled. The final katun in the Mayan calender—a twenty year sub-cycle that started in 1992 and will end in 2012—was prophesied to herald the Mayan return. This marks the entry into the "new solar age" and the dawning of the era of universal peace, fulfilling the promise of the Harmonic Convergence.

The Effects of the Harmonic Convergence

To understand the effects of the Harmonic Convergence, consider that everything in existence has its own field of resonance. Resonance describes the vibration or frequency rate at which a body of particles oscillates. Before the Harmonic Convergence, the Earth's field of resonance consistently measured at 7.8 Hertz. After the event, reports indicated an unprecedented change. Its characteristic readings of 7.8 Hz began to climb, reaching as high as 8.6 Hz, with unconfirmed reports declaring it to reach as high as 9.0 Hz. The change in resonance can be interpreted in a number of different ways, but the most significant of its meanings is crystal clear.

The shift is underway.

Using the Higher Vibration
to Achieve Radiant Health

You can use Earth's higher vibration to raise your vibration. In turn, this will expand your conscious awareness and open your heart, unearthing your darkest fears so you can face and overcome them, heal the Cartesian split and experience Radiant Health. The following explanations will help you understand how the process works.

At the basic level, both you and Earth act as electro-magnetic modules. Whenever two electric modules are placed in proximity to one another, the module with the lower frequency will attempt to raise its frequency to match that of the higher module. Because you are directly connected to Earth, as its frequency rises, you can raise your frequency to match it. Relative to your opportunity to achieve Radiant Health, maintaining a higher vibration enables you to break loose from dense vibratory patterns like fears, obsessions and dis-eases found in your emotional, mental and physical bodies.

However, human beings are endowed with free will, so being in constant proximity to Earth and its higher vibratory rate does not automatically ensure an increase in your vibratory rate.

You must make a conscious decision to raise your vibration.

Water, Vibration and Information

The water (H_2O) analogy further explains how the process of vibration works. Fill a small container with water and put it in a freezer. As the water freezes its molecular vibratory rate decreases and the liquid becomes solid. The H_2O molecules are now moving at a lower/slower rate of vibration, and they have access to only a very small area.

The area represents information.

Now, remove the ice from the freezer and place it on a flat surface. As the ice begins to thaw its vibration rate increases, the dense matter becomes lighter, and the H_2O covers a greater surface area.

The increase in vibration enables the H_2O to access even more area—information.

Add heat to the H_2O, and its vibration rate increases so much that the water turns to vaporous gas, expanding to cover its largest area. Increase your vibration rate and you can access more information. Put the information into action and it gives birth to experience, which ultimately leads to knowledge and increases your opportunity to discover your true nature.

This is the way to Radiant Health.

After making the decision to raise your vibration, use conscious breathing exercise #1—outlined in Chapter 4—and repeat the phrase "raise my vibration." As your vibration rises, you will feel a tingling sensation throughout your body, and the emotional calmness and peace of mind you will experience will validate that your vibration has been raised.

Science confirms that a relationship does indeed exist between one's rate of vibration and health or dis-ease. Love produces a very high frequency, while fear produces a substantially lower frequency. The lower your vibration, the more vulnerable you are to experience dis-ease. The higher your vibration, the stronger your resistance, and the greater your chance to experience Radiant Health.

Naadi Prophecies

You are now familiar with Hopi, Lakota, Mayan and Jewish prophecy concerning the importance of the current historical time period, prophesied events that have come to pass and the potential implications of those that are yet to be realized. However, even with an exceptional superhuman and Spiritual effort it would seem virtually impossible to overcome the monumental obstacles and challenges we face on a personal and global scale. Fortunately, God saw to it that if you sought refuge in the Divine you would be well protected during these most difficult times.

Just as Jewish prophets declared the coming of the Messiah, the birth of an Avatar, Sathya Sai Baba, was also prophesied. Fifty-six hundred years ago the great Rishis—wise men of ancient India, including Bhrugu, Vasishta, Agasty and Shuka, among others—foretold the entire future of mankind. Naadi is the collective name given to the prophetic manuscripts written by these sages. Today, the Naadi Granthas (Granthas means volumes) are held in safe-keeping by Sanskrit scholars and can be found in various parts of India. The ancient manuscripts, inscribed on palm leaves, are said to contain the full names and exact familial history (past, present and future) and characteristic of every human being that has lived, is living and will live on Earth.

The name of Avatar Sathya Sai Baba is found in the manuscripts.

In fact, the ancient manuscripts allude to a "Trinity of the Sai incarnations." Specifically, the manuscripts state that Avatar Sathya Sai Baba is the reincarnation of Sai Baba of Shirdi, and when the current life concludes, He will again incarnate as Prema Sai Baba. Sai Baba of Shirdi was the first of the "Sai Incarnations, was born in 1838 and left the planet on October 15, 1918."

After an eight-year intermission, Sathya Sai Baba, the second of the three Avatars, took birth.

An Avatar Is Born in India

In the early nineteen hundreds, the rural village of Puttaparthi in the state of Andhra Pradesh, India, was virtually unknown. The village contained less than one hundred people and the region was best known for its deadly population of scorpions and king cobras.

In the years to follow all that would change.

On November 23, 1926, an event took place in Puttaparthi that, in the coming years, would draw people from throughout the world, and make the tiny remote village and the Ashram contained within it, Prashanthi Nilayam, Abode of Peace, household names.

The event was the birth of an Avatar, Sathya Sai Baba.

What Is an Avatar?

According to Sanskrit scholars, the word *Avatar* means "Direct Incarnation of God." It is said that an Avatar incarnates—takes human form—during periods in which humanity has lost the path of virtue and is in danger of falling into total darkness— ignorance.

An Avatar has one purpose: the restoration of Dharma—right conduct, right action.

Unlike a highly evolved Spiritual teacher or even a master, an Avatar is born All-Knowing and Fully Realized. He is omniscient, omnipresent and omnipotent; born with complete awareness that He is connected to everything, exists in everything and is God Itself.

An Avatar is the Divine in human form.

The power, abilities and actions of an Avatar are extremely difficult to comprehend. To the untrained eye or unrealized person, He looks like any other human being. However, an Avatar has great power, which includes the ability to minimize, transmute or completely wipe out your Karma by direct intervention. Karma, the universal law of cause and effect, follows you from lifetime to lifetime and is simply stated by the phrase, "As you sow so shall you reap." By a mere look, being in His presence, or praying sincerely for God's grace, your Karma can be reduced or eliminated.

An Avatar, being a direct incarnation of the Tao, receives all prayers regardless of the name of God, Saint or deity to which the prayer is directed. This is an underlying beauty in the mission of an Avatar; regardless of whether your prayers are directed to Quan Yin, Buddha, Allah, Jesus, Krisna, Mother Mary or another aspect of the Divine, they will be received and answered by the Avatar.

Prophecy about Sathya Sai Baba

The Naadi Shuka volume that describes the birth and life of the current Avatar, Sathya Sai Baba, consists of hundreds of palm leaf manuscripts detailing all that He will accomplish in this present life, including the events that are still to come. The Naadi Shuka states that His true work will take place after the spring of 1979, and indeed He has become more widely recognized since that time.

Prophecies about the Sathya Sai Baba incarnation include the following:

- His mission will be relieving the distressed. (To this end, Satya Sai Baba has spent His life attending to the poor and needy. Notable projects include the completion of a drinking water project that brought water to over 973 drought-stricken villages serving over 1.5 million people; two Super Specialty Hospitals—one in Puttaparthi, another in Bangalore—which offer specialized surgical procedures, including open-heart surgery, with all treatments completely free of charge.)

- He will propagate Dharma—right conduct, right action. (The Sathya Sai Institute for Higher Learning, established in many countries around the world, specializes in EHV—Education in Human Values—and educates children from Elementary through College free of charge. The Sathya Sai Trust is responsible for building, maintaining and growing of these facilities.

Sai Baba does not handle any money. All facilities are built without government resources or funding.)

- The place in which He resides will become a Holy Land—His glory will spread far and wide and many people will come to Him. (According to the *New York Times* article—page A-8, December, 1, 2002—Sai Baba has devotees from 178 countries.)

- He will be able to assume different forms and be seen in several places simultaneously. (There are quite literally hundreds of books that contain firsthand reports chronicling amazing experiences in which Baba has been seen simultaneously in several places at once and has directly intervened to save persons from harm, or appeared to offer assistance in times of need.)

- He will be an incarnation of Love—He will not be concerned with public opinion and will do only what is right.

- He was previously Sai Baba of Shirdi.

- His life will be for the good of mankind.

- When unrighteousness reaches its full proportion—according to the Shuka Naadi it now stands at three-fourths proportion—His full powers will come into play.

- His efforts to save the world will increase ten-fold at the time of Pralaya Kaala—the end of this world cycle.

The Mayan, Lakota, Hopi and Jewish prophecies also refer directly or indirectly to the end of this world cycle. At present, the Shuka Naadi proclaims that Sathya Sai Baba displays only one-tenth of His real self.

Prophecies also related to Sathya Sai Baba can be found in the works of Edgar Cayce and Nostradamus as well as in the Holy Bible—Book of Revelation—and the Koran—the Holy book of the Islamic faith.

The Avatar and Your Journey to Radiant Health

It is not important to believe.

It is important to take action—to put Love into Action.

Take a trip to Puttaparthi, India, and visit Prashanthi Nilayam and Sai Baba. Experience the Abode of Peace, the multi-cultural coming together of peoples from all over the world. Otherwise, take comfort in the fact that the Divine has come in human form specifically to assist the world through the upcoming shift, and you in realizing your true nature and becoming a blazing beacon of Love.

Prophetic Possibilities

Each of the previous prophecies was received by peoples from different cultures, lands and historical time periods. Yet all are being fulfilled in the current time period. And, even if the timing of their fulfillment might be considered coincidental, their message cannot. Although only a very small portion of prophecies were presented in this chapter, all concur that the world is heading towards a profound change. The critical question is—will the shift occur by means of anarchy or conscious revelation?

The decision is, in part, up to you.

The degree to which personal and collective hardship or ease will be experienced during the transformation is determined by the free will choices of all human beings. Taking human free will into consideration, each of the previous prophecies outlines two possible scenarios. One warns of a coming Armageddon—a final battle between the forces of good/Light and evil/Darkness that will either destroy the world, or all the evil in it. The other proposes an Apocalypse—traditionally defined as a revelation—which will serve to awaken humanity from its Spiritual hibernation. The Apocalypse phenomenon has already affected a great many individuals worldwide, and it continues to grow—see Section Seven. Now you can make the conscious decision to experience your own Apocalypse.

You can help prevent Armageddon.

Apply the seven steps to Radiant Health, and you consciously choose Apocalypse. Change your patterns from those that are associated with Darkness—fear, ignorance and destruction—to those that are connected to Light—love, wisdom and construction—and your energy will assist the collective consciousness of humanity in its shift from Darkness to Light.

The direction in which the pendulum will swing, in part, depends on your choices.

The decision is yours.

The time to act is now.

3

You, the World and Radiant Health

The life-affirming decision to embark on *The Journey to Radiant Health* marks the starting point of your change in consciousness. As a catalyst it will ignite your process of awakening, promoting greater personal conscious awareness.

Your decision makes it possible to snap out of the sleepwalking state of Maya, dispel the Darkness of fear and ignorance from your mind, and welcome the Light of love and harmony. When your path is illuminated with Light, it will be easier to trust the process of life and your own heart's intuitive impulses.

As the Light illuminates your consciousness it will propel you to live more fully in the present moment. This elevates your emotional, mental and physical health and vitality.

But there is so much more.

Your Decisions Impact Human Consciousness

Your decision to embark on *The Journey to Radiant Health* also supports humanity's movement towards the Light. Every conscious choice you make to bring more love and Light to your life brings more love and Light to everyone in your world. This is an important point to consider as the world struggles to free itself from the Darkness of a possible Armageddon.

The hectic pace of daily life can cause you to feel overwhelmed, making it difficult to devote your time and energy to causes that can have a positive impact on the world. But don't worry because regardless of how small or insignificant, every action that enables you to live in the Light of love and harmony brings light to the world. Even the simple choice to pray for peace and meditate on love can have a large enough impact to make the difference between Armageddon and Apocalypse.

Every human being is a thread that is intimately interwoven into the fabric of the collective consciousness. As such, your actions emit a wave of energy that affects every strand in its matrix. By being a container and dispenser of Light you can transmit the radiance of love, knowledge, truth and wisdom to every strand in the collective human consciousness.

One Man's Journey Illuminates His World

Many men in recorded history were considered great leaders; but among them only one had the fortitude to consciously step out of the Darkness and live in the Light. His story is a unique, compelling, and inspiring example of Spiritual potential fulfilled. His life clearly displays the power of the human Spirit to end a reign of tyranny, violence and destruction, embrace the supreme spiritual path—service to others—and carry it out by becoming a living example of the highest Spiritual principles—love and devotion.

His name was Asoka.

As his reign began he was known as *"Asoka the Cruel."*

In the third century B.C., at the apex of the Kali Yugas, Emperor Asoka rose to the height of his power. His kingdom stretched from Bengal in the east, to Afghanistan in the northwest, to Mysore in the south. Asoka knew that his legacy would be determined by his ability to complete the conquest of the Indian peninsula. Following in his father and grandfather's footsteps, Asoka invaded and conquered Kalinga.

Although he was victorious in battle, hundreds of thousands were killed, wounded and tortured. Viewing the carnage transformed Asoka and at the peak of his power, while still possessing the strength to continue his conquests, he made a conscious decision to turn away from war. In an unprecedented and stunning act of courage that has yet to be duplicated by any modern world leader, Asoka publicly expressed repentance for his actions, swearing never again to unsheathe his sword. He renounced war and violence, and devoted his full attention to the study, practice and promotion of Dharma—right action and right conduct. As he changed, so did the name previously attached to him.

Asoka came to be known as *"The Beloved of the Gods."*

Emperor Asoka wished non-violence, self-control and the practice of serenity and mildness for all beings. He desired that his sons and grandsons only think of conquest by piety. Asoka's indoctrination into selfless service and non-violence empowered him to establish a government founded on these principles. Asoka became a devoted ruler of high moral character modeling, among others, the qualities of honesty, integrity, self-sacrifice, kindness, patience and harmony as he served those he ruled.

Asoka's actions are a blueprint for individual, societal and planetary Radiant Health. Not by preaching, but by loving and mindful actions, Asoka became a beacon of Light in a world of Darkness. The courage he displayed by becoming a man of peace in a world saturated with violence provides us with hope for a brighter today and a better tomorrow.

Bringing Radiant Health to Your World

You do not have to be an emperor to make a difference in the world. Focus first on healing yourself and your actions will effect healing elsewhere. The smile you give, the helping hand you extend or the time you take to listen advances the cause of healing and brings Radiant Health to your world. Every moment that you spend in conscious awareness infuses the world with more love and Light. Every wound that you heal brings more healing to the world. Every prayer you pray and every moment you pause to meditate brings the promise of world peace and harmony a step close to realization. Every song, smile and laugh that rises from your heart radiates love and Light to the world.

And the world needs your Light.

The Light raises your vibration and has the power to affect others. It provides others with an opportunity to identify and dispel their own Darkness. Your efforts to embody qualities of love such as forgiveness, patience, courage, trust, compassion, acceptance, peace and humility enable others to open their hearts and experience their own Apocalypse. Eventually, love will push Armageddon totally out of the realm of possibility.

Every thought, feeling, or action that rises from the heart plants a seed. Even if the seeds do not immediately take root, at some point they will germinate. Just keep planting seeds until they sprout. Eventually they will grow strong enough to bear fruit. As the seeds take root, those who have been affected by your Light and love will feel inspired and motivated to welcome the Light of love into their own hearts and minds.

The Bridge to Conscious Awareness

Crossing the bridge to conscious awareness is a prerequisite on *The Journey to Radiant Health*. The bridge will establish your foothold on the path to Radiant Health by planting you on the shore of conscious awareness. Its seven steps can help dispel the effects of Darkness and fear from your heart and mind, provide you with a fresh perspective on life and make your journey a little easier.

Step 1: Accept pain, difficulties, challenges and obstacles as being a natural part of life.

Step 2: Identify and acknowledge—to yourself, others and God— your fears, difficulties, challenges and obstacles.

Step 3: Regardless of the challenges, fears, obstacles or difficulties you might face, do not stop, turn back or give up in your search for peace.

Step 4: Accept yourself just as you are. Work to master your ego and fears, but do not judge yourself for having them.

Step 5: View everyone and everything in your life as an instrument sent by Spirit to help you find and clear away the impurities that keep you from finding lasting contentment.

Step 6: Share all of your experiences—the happiness and sorrow, joy and pain—with those that love and support you.

Step 7: Seek to serve others from a heart filled with love and joy.

SECTION TWO

On average, you breathe about 21,600 times a day, which gives you plenty of opportunities to increase your self-awareness.

-4-

Conscious Breathing:
A Path to Self-Awareness

*Conscious breathing is the vehicle that brings us
back to the present moment and keeps us here.*
—Thich Nhat Hanh

Learn to live in the moment and follow your heart (rather than your mind) and you will experience Radiant Health. For thousands of years, a simple technique has existed that will enable you to get out of the mind and into the heart. The technique has the power to keep your focus and attention in the here and now. It is employed by Yogis, sages and other beings that walk the path of self-awareness.

The technique is conscious breathing.

Conscious breathing facilitates the process of awakening by enhancing your conscious awareness. The breath, like everything in nature, moves in rhythmic cycles, expanding and contracting. Everyone is born on an inhale and expires on an exhale, and because breath is the gateway to experiences, everything received on an in breath can be released on an out breath. Because breathing is not given much thought or attention and is, for the most part, involuntary, the power of conscious breathing to effect change remains largely unrecognized. Conscious breathing, however, provides you a simple and direct method by which to turn your focus and attention inward and access Spirit. For this reason conscious breathing is the starting point and foundation on *The Journey to Radiant Health*.

The benefits of conscious breathing are unique. Buddhists say that conscious breathing is the most effective tool to train the mind and develop focus. With consistent practice, conscious breathing will assist you to recognize and detach from reactive thoughts and emotions. In this way, conscious breathing can help keep you emotionally centered and mentally clear, thereby reducing the dis-ease-producing effects of stress and tension.

The Power of Conscious Breathing

For thousands of years, many Spiritual-based, self-awareness-raising practices such as meditation, Yoga, Chi-Gong and martial arts have taught the importance of being able to regulate the breath. The ability to regulate the functions of the body, mind and emotions exerts a positive influence on your Spiritual growth. Controlling the breath enables you to control the mind, emotions and vital functions of the body.

On average, you breathe about 21,600 times a day, which gives you plenty of opportunities to increase your self-awareness. Conscious breathing also can increase energy, release emotions, facilitate physical healing and restore overall balance. On a more esoteric level, the use of conscious breathing and meditation techniques expands your awareness to the point where the ego dissolves. Then you consciously experience your connection to everything in existence.

Typically, it is unusual to be taught anything about breathing. Even rarer are classes that teach breathing techniques and their effects. Respiration, however, accounts for approximately 80% of your energy. How you breathe is as important to your emotional and mental well-being as it is to your physical health. Often, a traumatic event must occur before appreciating the importance of breathing. Yet, nothing will snap you back into the moment quicker than losing your breath or having respiratory trouble. When breathing becomes difficult, you are brought face to face with your physical mortality. Anything that might have been important becomes insignificant relative to catching your breath.

Asthma is an example of a physical breathing affliction that also has mental and emotional implications. In purely physical terms, asthma is a respiratory problem resulting from a restriction of the bronchial walls that makes breathing difficult. It is directly related to overexertion of the lungs usually caused by excessive exercise, air pollution, tobacco smoke, common allergens, or dehydration (often a glass of water can alleviate an asthma attack).

Pharmaceutical products might provide temporary relief from the symptoms of asthma, but they do nothing to uncover, address or heal the core issue of the dis-ease. From a holistic viewpoint, an approach that encompasses all aspects of the self would better serve to facilitate a complete recovery. For example, emotions like unresolved grief, sadness, anxiety, low self-esteem or feeling smothered by parents or authority figures can trigger an asthma attack. Stress and toxic thoughts are also associated with asthmatic reactions. When a holistic approach is taken to healing, the dis-ease is less likely to reappear. A holistic approach to healing dis-ease, which includes conscious breathing as its foundation, can bring hidden, repressed or denied emotions and thoughts to the surface for examination, expression and release.

Increasing awareness, as a direct result of conscious breathing, also increases the likelihood that the core issues will rise to the surface. Although it might not be wise to throw out the inhaler immediately, by identifying and working through the mental and emotional causes of asthma, the medicine cabinet might be opened one day only to find the inhaler collecting dust.

Getting into Action

Now that you are aware of the benefits of conscious breathing, it is time to get into action. Observation is key to the first conscious breathing exercise. You can make this initial exercise easier by adding the qualities of willingness, introspection and perseverance to your practice. Willingness enables you to keep an open mind. Introspection keeps your focus and attention turned inward, enabling you to ignore external distractions and observe and release any thoughts, emotions or sensations that arise during your practice. Perseverance will move you through obstacles when they appear, or when the practice becomes mundane. Use the guidelines below to set up your initial practice.

1. Set aside five to ten minutes each morning, afternoon and evening to practice the exercise.

2. Create a quiet space to practice the exercise and remove your shoes.

3. Sit on a chair and support your back with a pillow in order to keep your spine straight. Place your feet flat on the floor and place your hands in your lap, palms facing up.

4. If the position causes physical pain, then find a comfortable position. If necessary, lie flat to do the exercise.

5. Close your eyes, or softly gaze at the tip of your nose.

CONSCIOUS BREATHING EXERCISE #1
THE ANNAPANA TECHNIQUE

1. Keep your posture and spine straight, chin parallel with the ground.

2. Focus on the area between the top of your upper lip and the entrance to your nasal passages.

3. Without changing your breathing, become aware of the inhales and the exhales.

4. Observe the breath.

If sitting straight with the spine erect is unfamiliar, it might feel a bit uncomfortable. It is important to maintain an erect spine because it allows energy to flow unobstructed from the brain through the spinal column to the organs, muscles and tissues. Think of the spine like a telephone cord; a crooked line causes static, reduces the flow of energy and transmits incomplete or unclear messages. A straight line moves energy in a quick, efficient and clear manner. Sitting straight decompresses the spine and creates more length. Length translates into space and space translates into comfort. As your body gets used to the posture it will become more relaxed and comfortable, and you might notice yourself becoming more alert, energized and refreshed.

The practice begins by becoming aware of your breathing. Notice the texture. Is it choppy or smooth, deep or shallow, erratic or fluid? Do not judge it. Keep your focus on the area between the rings of the nasal passages and the upper lip. As the practice becomes familiar and comfortable, increase your practice time.

This conscious breathing exercise has a two-fold purpose. First, it will help you relax. As the body relaxes, stress is reduced and tension melts away. Second, it increases self-awareness and builds discipline. Keeping your attention and focus on the breath keeps you in the present moment. When thoughts or emotions distract you, simply return your focus to the breath. This exercise will help you develop and strengthen your focus, but be aware that it takes time to build a strong and solid foundation. So be moderate. This is a step-by-step process.

If your commitment wanes or fluctuates simply recommit to your practice and remember, easy does it. Accept where you are, otherwise you run the risk of sabotaging your efforts or quitting altogether. This is the first of five conscious breathing exercises and its purpose is to help you focus on the breath, not master it. Mastery comes with time and practice. Each exercise is progressive, but you can always return to review. Listed below are some tips to keep in mind while you practice.

1. Do not rush. Progress comes with practice.

2. Be willing to acknowledge and overcome obstacles that impede your progress. This might include wandering thoughts like "I wonder if Sally is going to call," "How much time do I have left?" or "I should be studying." It also might include feeling uncomfortable emotions like frustration, impatience and anxi-

ety. Also acknowledge distractions to your practice such as "I do not have enough time," "I do not see any progress" or "This is too difficult."

3. Keep in mind that the practice is designed to increase your self-awareness, not to be perfect in the practice.

4. Reinforce your practice with positive affirmations such as "I am doing a good job in this moment" or "I am willing to practice today."

5. Use a journal to keep track of your progress. Answer the following questions:

   • Did any feelings, thoughts or noises distract me?
   • Did I hold my breath?
   • Did I lose consciousness—fall asleep?

-5-

Fundamental
Breathing Patterns

The way most people breathe is characterized by one of four fundamental patterns. Each pattern is unique in form and function. The first, automatic breathing, is a function of the autonomic nervous system (ANS) and requires no conscious effort to sustain. The second, archetypal breathing, is a common breathing pattern learned through your life experiences. The third, diaphragmatic breathing, is the closest pattern to conscious breathing, but lacks its most important features. The fourth, conscious breathing, increases your conscious awareness and makes Radiant Health attainable. A study of the first three will expose their ineffectiveness in helping you increase your awareness and achieve Radiant Health.

Automatic Breathing

Breathing is a function controlled by the autonomic nervous system. If you do not pay attention to your breathing, the ANS will automatically furnish you with breath throughout your life. Because automatic breathing needs no conscious effort on your part to direct, it can be considered the breath of survival.

However, it is unstable, and here is why.

The sympathetic and parasympathetic nervous systems form the foundation of the ANS and automatic breathing. The parasympathetic nervous system is in charge of conserving energy. It is active when you are calm, keeping your breathing balanced, steady and unwavering. The sympathetic nervous system is responsible for activating your energy. It takes over when you become upset or disturbed, inducing the fight or flight reaction. The sympathetic nervous system causes adrenaline and other hormones and chemicals to be released into the body to prepare you to handle the disturbance.

There are instances in which the sympathetic nervous system reaction is important and necessary. For example, in a crisis you might need the superhuman strength adrenaline provides to save a life. However, in an instant, an activated sympathetic nervous system can undermine your focus and clarity. ANS breathing can cause you to involuntarily react to your environment. React and you ride the roller coaster of mental and emotional ups and downs, including physiological changes. Sleepless nights are just one of many insidious afflictions that result from mental or emotional upsets.

Conscious Breathing Counteracts Harmful Sympathetic Nervous System Effects

Conscious breathing can counter the harmful effects of the sympathetic nervous system. Conscious breathing enables you to manage your emotional and mental energies, preventing the sympathetic nervous system from being activated and enabling you to detach from dis-ease-producing thoughts and emotions like obsessions, rage and guilt. You will find detachment exercises in Chapters 21 and 27. The bottom line is that automatic breathing is not an effective breathing pattern for increasing self-awareness.

On the other hand, the first conscious breathing exercise taught you how to become aware of your breathing. The second technique will teach you how to control your breath, and how to use it to manage your physical, mental and emotional energy. Then, instead of being subject to the reactive potential of your sympathetic nervous system, conscious breathing can be implemented when your mental clarity and emotional stability are challenged.

Archetypal Breathing

A baby's breath flows free. As it inhales, its belly expands and fills completely with breath. As the baby exhales, its belly naturally and gently collapses. The effects of physical, mental and emotional trauma cause this initial breathing pattern to change. The open and natural pattern of deep abdominal breathing that a baby enjoys is abandoned. The breath moves into the chest and shallow breathing becomes the norm. The change occurs, as a conscious or subconscious mechanism, to protect you from feeling the raw and sometimes overwhelmingly intense emotions associated with life's more painful and traumatic experiences. In a figurative way, layers of armor are constructed around the heart as a means of protection from emotional, mental or physical pain.

Hiding pain is at the core of the second fundamental breathing pattern, archetypal breathing.

Archetypal breathing, as it relates to health, ostensibly encourages good posture. The archetypal breathing method consists of sucking in the gut, straightening the spine and sticking out the chest. The emphasis is on how one looks, rather than how one feels. Archetypal breathing is identified by key features associated with clavicular breathing; the breath is shallow, reaching only the upper regions of the torso. Contrary to a natural and relaxed state of breathing where the abdomen is the first area to be filled on the inhale and the chest is the last, the archetypal breathing model immediately inflates the chest and the abdomen receives little or no air.

Inflating the chest and sucking in the gut is not a natural breathing pattern.

It is unhealthy because it uses only a small fraction—typically 12%—of your lung capacity. Also, because the abdomen is sucked in on the inhale, vital life force energy is diminished, resulting in lower resistance to dis-ease. Natural, fluid breathing takes air into the pear-shaped lungs, inflating them completely from bottom to top. In terms of holistic health, however, it is important to note that the shallow chest-inflating archetypal breathing disassociates you from your feelings.

The shallower your breath, the less you feel.

The Roots of Archetypal Breathing

Disseminated in physical education classes, military training and mainstream media messages, archetypal breathing promotes style over substance. The archetypal breathing method teaches both men and women to breathe into the chest and suck in the abdomen on the inhale.

As men breathe into the chest and suck in the gut on the inhale, they create an external appearance of strength. Appearances, however, can be deceiving. To maintain the appearance of strength, men are led to believe that they have to withhold tenderness because it can be misconstrued as weakness. Withholding emotions like sadness, grief and pain in order to maintain an appearance of strength actually compromises it. In fact, withholding emotions promotes emotional and mental rigidity, which eventually leads to physical dis-ease.

The true measure of strength in a man is found in his ability to express the truth with love and compassion.

As women breathe into the chest and tuck in the tummy on the inhale, they create an image of beauty. To maintain the image of beauty, women are led to believe that they have to withhold the truth because standing for truth can make them appear hostile. Withholding truth, however, compromises a woman's emotional and mental well-being and can jeopardize her physical health, especially when it prohibits her from taking a stand, for herself or others. Withholding the truth can cause a woman to allow herself to be abused.

The true measure of beauty in a woman is related to her ability to express love that is grounded in truth.

Image has nothing to do with love. We are not being true to ourselves when we try to maintain an image. While archetypal breathing builds layers of armor around the heart, conscious breathing builds a foundation that dissolves the armor and opens the heart. Conscious breathing makes mental, emotional and physical health and well-being the central focus.

Diaphragmatic Breathing

The third pattern, diaphragmatic breathing, is a step closer to conscious breathing in that it requires a conscious effort to bring the breath into the diaphragm. The diaphragm is located just below the breastbone or sternum on the chest.

Diaphragmatic breathing, also known as intercostal or middle breathing, steps beyond archetypal breathing. It draws the breath deeper into the body, reaching as far as the solar plexus. Often used by performing artists, diaphragmatic/intercostal breathing is much better for the physical body than ANS or archetypal breathing. Diaphragmatic breathing, by using a greater portion of the lungs' total capacity, brings more oxygen to the blood stream.

Diaphragmatic breathing pushes the diaphragm down on the inhale. This action massages the internal organs. As the diaphragm moves up during the exhale, it massages the heart. These actions stimulate the internal organs—helping them to function more efficiently and effectively. They are the most outstanding health-producing qualities attributed to diaphragmatic breathing. Still, middle breathing is a pattern that lacks the ability to increase conscious awareness and promote Radiant Health.

Choosing the Proper Breathing Method

Prana is a Sanskrit word that means "life force energy." Prana exists in air, water, food, the atmospheric ethers and every living particle found in the universe. Although science has not yet been able to identify prana, it is known by sages to be the energy responsible for healing the physical body during sleep.

Conscious Breathing and Prana

Conscious breathing is the only known breathing method capable of drawing in prana and distributing it throughout the body. After conscious breathing has saturated the body with prana, reserves are stored in the medulla to be used when a boost of life force energy is needed—in times of crisis or stress, emotional upheaval or mental fatigue. Your breathing habits directly affect the amount of prana you are able to extract from the air and ethers. Of the four fundamental breathing patterns, only conscious breathing enables you to extract prana directly from the ethers and bring it into your body for immediate use, or store it for future use.

Characterized by deep abdominal breathing, conscious breathing is the most effective breathing method for taking in oxygen and prana. Conscious breathing also rids the body of toxic waste, releases repressed emotions, facilitates mental focus and clarity and heals physical injuries. The healing attributes of deep abdominal breathing which are inherent in conscious breathing can propel you to Radiant Health. The following illuminates the details.

The Effects of Conscious Breathing

When breathing into the abdomen, the lungs are filled to capacity and the blood receives the greatest amounts of oxygen and prana.

Detailed in conscious breathing exercise #3 (page 56), the ratio of exhale to inhale enables you to expel more toxic carbon dioxide from the blood.

While oxygen will keep the body alive, prana heals the body and can make it incorruptible.[1] Conscious breathing is distinguished by nasal passage breathing because prana can only be received through the nasal passages.

Deep abdominal breathing is the most effective method for consistent stimulation of the lymphatic system. Blood is pumped through the body by the heart, but the lymphatic system relies on breathing or exercise to stimulate it. To get an idea of the lymphatic system's importance, consider this: if it were to shut down, you would die within 24 hours. Breathing deeply into the abdomen fully activates the lymphatic system and can increase its detoxification rate up to 15 times higher than normal.

On the inhale, the diaphragm moves down, the abdomen expands, the internal organs are massaged and any stagnant energy in the organs is expelled.

As the internal organs are stimulated, they function more efficiently and effectively.

The internal organs regulate healthy and unhealthy emotions and thought patterns. During deep abdominal conscious breathing, toxic dis-ease-producing emotions or thoughts that have become lodged in the psychosomatic cellular structure rise to the surface. After they have been identified, they can be healed and released.

On the exhale, the abdomen contracts and the diaphragm moves up, massaging the heart. Any stagnant emotional energy lodged in the metaphysical cellular structure known as the heart can rise to the surface, be examined, healed and released.

Conscious breathing develops greater focus. The mind is trained by the act of conscious breathing to focus on one task.

As the psychosomatic cellular structure is balanced and harmonized the Cartesian split will heal, providing emotional, mental and physical integration.

The navel area is where clairvoyants say the soul is housed. As the conscious breathing brings the breath deep into the abdomen, the soul can be aroused from its waking slumber and your life's purpose can be identified.

By using meditation and abdominal breathing in conjunction, oxygen and prana can be directed to the location of an injury, helping to facilitate physical healing. The breath can be visualized passing through the nasal passages and being drawn into the injured or dis-eased muscles, organs, bones or tissues. You can also add a soothing, healing or favorite color, or find the one that is appropriate to your condition and healing needs. See "Colors: Their Meanings and Uses" and "The Chakra Systems" in the Appendix.

The Importance of Breathing through the Nostrils

One of the most important facets of conscious breathing is using only the nostrils to breathe. The nostrils purify air by filtering out pollutants and other irritants. Mouth breathing dries out its mucus membranes and the mouth has no filters to remove pollutants, bacteria or germs.

Breathing through the nasal passages enables you to regulate the breath by drawing it in fully and slowly. This process enables you to use the full capacity of your lungs to direct your breath into the tense areas in the body. Nasal passage breathing increases the amount of prana brought into the body, because prana enters the body through the olfactory organs (which reside at the back of the nasal passages) not the mouth. Prana passes through the olfactory organs into the medulla—the hind part of the vertebrate brain. From there it is taken to the central nervous system and brain, where it charges the electroprotonic center of every cell in the body. Breathing through the nasal passages also enables you to breathe in a consistent, rhythmic and fluid pattern of inhales and exhales.

There are a several ways to move breath through the nostrils. The most common is to sniff the air in through the entrance of the nasal passages. Another is to expand the nostrils and snort the breath in through the open nostrils. Rather than sniffing or snorting, draw the breath through the nostrils, to the back of the throat, on the inhale. Drawing the breath into the back of the throat creates a sound similar to the sound emitted by someone who is deep in sleep. When exhaling—also through the nostrils—let the breath pass through the throat, closing the esophagus slightly, and allow the same sound to be emitted from the back of the throat.

Because conscious breathing trains the mind to stay focused on a singular task, wandering thoughts can be kept to a minimum. With practice, it will become easier to return your focus and attention to your breath when it drifts. Conscious breathing also makes it easier to remain emotionally centered and mentally clear regardless of the pressure or intensity in any situation.

7

The Final Four Exercises

CONSCIOUS BREATHING EXERCISE #2

Practice this exercise for five to ten minutes each morning, afternoon and evening. Choose a comfortable, quiet place to practice. Try to select consistent practice times; and as in the previous exercise, remove your shoes, sit on a chair and support your back with a pillow. Keep your spine erect and place your hands in your lap with the palms facing up. Put your feet flat on the floor and begin.

1. Take a few deep breaths. Relax your shoulders, neck and back.

2. Slowly draw in the breath from the back of the nasal passages, at the back of the throat. Draw the breath deep into the abdomen and let the abdomen expand as you inhale.

3. When the abdomen reaches full capacity immediately, without holding the breath, begin to exhale slowly and completely, letting the abdomen collapse towards the spine.

4. Regulate the breath. Keep the cycle of inhales and exhales consistent by inhaling and exhaling to the same count. For example, if your inhale ends at the count of six, then exhale to the count of six.

5. Work to lengthen the breath. Focus on breathing as slowly and deeply as possible. Extend the abdomen out as far as possible on the inhale and collapse it as far back to the spine as possible on the exhale.

Conscious breathing exercise #2 will help you modify, lengthen and control your breathing. It also helps you practice using the full capacity of the lungs by expanding and contracting the abdomen. More importantly, because the focus of the inhale is at the back of the nasal passages rather than the entrance, this conscious breathing exercise draws in prana. By focusing on drawing the breath in at the back of the nasal passages, it also makes nasal passage breathing easier for those who suffer from blocked sinuses. Although it takes time, effort and patience to perfect, drawing the breath in will become easier and more effective. If breathing exclusively through the nostrils is new, you might initially experience feelings such as anxiety or discomfort.

This is not unusual.

It is a temporary condition that will diminish and, with continued practice, eventually disappear. If you experience anxiety, try to relax. Give yourself some time to adjust. The transition from archetypal, automatic or diaphragmatic breathing to conscious breathing takes practice. If you need to breathe through the mouth, do so—just close the mouth for longer and longer periods during your practice. As your conscious breathing practice becomes more familiar, you will feel more comfortable.

The Challenges of Shifting to Conscious Breathing

There are two common challenges associated with conscious breathing. The first is being able to draw the breath deep into the abdomen. At the outset it can feel awkward, especially considering that you have spent most of your life breathing shallowly or into the upper chest. It takes some time and effort to get used to expanding the abdomen on the inhale and collapsing it on the exhale.

Until you become accustomed to taking deep, full breaths into the abdomen, try to relax the chest on the inhale. In other words, make a conscious effort to keep the breath from moving the chest. If the chest continues to expand and lift on the inhale, place the left

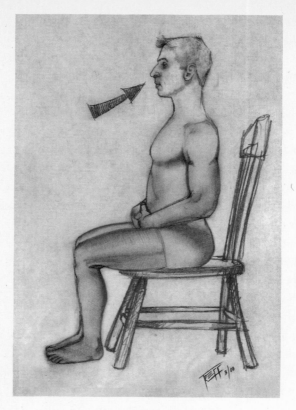

ILLUSTRATION #1. The inhale
Note the hand placement and abdomen extension

hand on the abdomen with the thumb on or just below the belly
button. The bottom edge of the left hand should rest on or near the
top of the pubic bone. Place the right hand on top of the left hand.
Relax the body as much as possible. Close your eyes, and on the
inhale allow the abdomen to push your hands out.

The second challenge is to let go of the thinking that accompanies the initial phase of the practice. The mind, in an attempt to
figure out the technique, will try to control the practice. The result is
that you will find yourself thinking about breathing into the abdo-

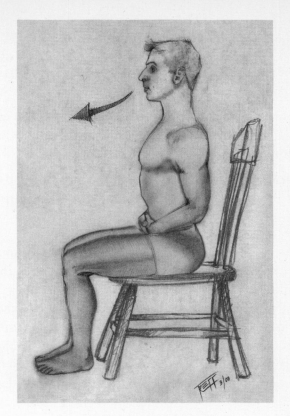

ILLUSTRATION #2. The exhale
Note the collapsing of the abdomen

men, but actually breathing into the chest. Rather than letting the mind control the practice, trust the body to remember its natural breathing pattern. As you relax the body will return to the natural breathing pattern of a baby.

When the abdomen is full, exhale the breath slowly, allowing the abdomen to collapse towards the spine. See illustration #2. Keep your hands over the abdomen and as you exhale and the abdomen deflates, use the hands as a guide to gently push the abdomen toward the spine.

CONSCIOUS BREATHING EXERCISE #3

1. Slowly draw the breath in through the back of the nasal passages and count until the inhale is complete.

2. Exhale the breath slowly, doubling the count of the inhale. For example, if you inhale to the count of six, then exhale slow enough to reach the count of twelve.

3. Complete two rounds a day, one in the morning and evening. Sixteen breaths (complete inhales and exhales) comprise one round.

This exercise floods the body with prana, which promotes physical healing, mental acuity and emotional stability. Each inhale draws prana into the body, the most powerful substance for rejuvenating cells. Slow inhales fully oxygenate the system. Slow exhales stimulate the lymphatic system and release more carbon dioxide. The more oxygen and prana drawn into the cells, the more they become supercharged with energy. The more the lymphatic system is stimulated, the more toxins that can be eliminated from the body.

CONSCIOUS BREATHING EXERCISE #4

1. When you awaken, take a slow, deep breath into the abdomen.

2. On the exhale, gently pull your knees to your chest.

3. On the next slow inhale, release the knees and gently stretch your arms above your head.

4. On the exhale, massage any tense or stiff areas of the body.

5. Offer a prayer of gratitude to God for two things that make you feel grateful to be alive.

6. Set a *clear* intention for the day such as: "I will focus on breathing," "I will be of service" or "I will be calm and patient."

7. Get out of bed and stretch gently in conjunction with the breath—expand on the inhales and contract on the exhales.

This three to five minute exercise provides tremendous benefits. Breathing deep into the abdomen stimulates the internal organs and expels toxins. Pulling the knees close to the chest contracts the abdomen and stretches the lower back, releasing tension. Stretching the arms over the head opens the lungs. Massaging the body increases warmth, circulation and blood flow. What you think of at the moment you awake sets the tone for your day. Offering a prayer of gratitude puts the mind in a positive frame, which is a great way to start your day. A clear intention gives you a starting point on which to focus. When you set an intention first thing in the morning, you are likely to see it materialize at some point during the course of the day.

CONSCIOUS BREATHING EXERCISE #5

1. Find a quiet place in nature and sit comfortably or lie flat on your back.

2. Breathe slowly and deeply, consciously releasing all thoughts and emotions.

3. Concentrate on *feeling* your connection to Mother Earth and Father Sky.

4. Breathe slowly and expand your awareness beyond your body.

5. Try to *connect with* the consciousness that exists in the plants, animals and trees.

This esoteric conscious breathing exercise will help you *extend* your awareness beyond the self. Here, you are working to experience your interdependent connection with everything in nature, the world and the universe. Do not worry if you do not feel the connection right away. It takes time and practice to become sensitive to the

life force that exists in all things. If you practice consistently, do not be
surprised if you begin to get messages from the beings in nature—trees
animals, mountains, birds or waters.

Everything in the universe, whether it is classified as animate or inani-
mate, contains consciousness. Be consistent in your practice and you will
become more sensitive to the life force energy that exists in you and
everything around you.

Taking a conscious breath is an opportunity to be here now.

A conscious breath is a return to simplicity, a chance to slow down
and feel, to taste life's sweet nectar and savor its beauty. A conscious
breath can give you a new perspective and keep you from getting swept
away by the fast moving currents of modern life. Conscious breathing
provides you with an opportunity to awaken from the spell of Maya, cast
off her chains and experience the awakened state of Radiant Health.

To breathe is to feel and to feel is to heal.

SECTION THREE

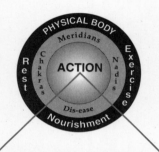

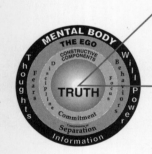

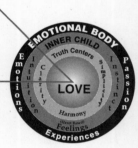

SACRED TRINITY
OF
RADIANT HEALTH

8

The Sacred Trinity
of Radiant Health

Say not, "I have found the truth,"
but say rather, "I have found a truth."
Say not, "I have found the path of the soul."
Say rather, "I have met the soul walking upon my path."
For the soul walks upon all paths.
The soul walks not upon a line,
neither does it grow like a reed.
The soul unfolds itself, like a lotus of countless petals.
—Kahlil Gibran, The Prophet

A flower unfolds petal by petal to reveal its whole beauty and the same can be said about you. Like God's most precious, beautiful and fragrant flower, you are a glorious composition containing many parts. The first part of the flower is the petals. Each petal represents a particular of your personality, including all your thoughts and emotions. With love, the flower blossoms, the petals open and the center, which contains your soul, is revealed. The soul is the second part of the flower, the individualized part of God that you represent. There is, however, one more part of the flower. It is the most pure, wholesome and important part and yet is the most difficult to find. It is invisible to the naked eye and yet the entire universe is contained within it.

The third and final part is called Spirit.

The Spirit is completely untouched and unaffected by anything that the personality experiences and expresses. The Spirit is the absolute perfect essence and expression of God. The seven steps on *The Journey to Radiant Health* are specifically intended to give you direct contact and a direct experience of God, your Spirit.

God is Love. God is Light.

Your true nature is that of Love and Light.

Practice the steps consciously, faithfully and with determination and you will move beyond Darkness, extinguish the ego and fear and experience the part of your true nature which is beyond time and space.

Each step on *The Journey to Radiant Health* will bring you closer to the ultimate unfolding, until the moment arrives when you experience the effulgent joy and fulfillment of being fully present in the here and now. To know, in truth, that you are Spirit and to see the same Spirit that you are in everyone and everything.

Bliss is unending joy that you feel when you experience total awareness.

To get to the essence, Spirit, you first have to identify and move beyond the various petals of your personality. These petals, based in ego, keep you from recognizing your soul, experiencing your Spirit and realizing your inherent beauty and perfection. Increase your awareness and you create an opportunity to move into the heart.

Your heart is part of the interwoven tapestry that opens the path to your soul, which in turn connects you to Spirit—everyone and everything in existence. However, this can only be realized experientially. When it is, the illusion of separation, including the thoughts and emotions that accompany the illusion such as emptiness, loneliness, discontentment, anxiety, boredom, confusion, anger or turmoil, will be dispelled. Raising your conscious awareness makes it easier to access the heart, realize your true beauty and embrace your Divine perfection. Living in your heart enables you to realize the Divine beauty and perfection of every petal of the personality, and still work to move beyond them.

The Sacred Trinity of Radiant Health is a dynamic model comprised of the three bodies: emotional, mental and physical. The emotional body expresses feminine energy, the mental body expresses masculine energy and the physical body expresses the energy of the Divine Child—the integration of feminine and masculine energy. The Sacred Trinity has two functions, and each will enable you to explore the petals of your personality.

The first is its basic function.

The second is its esoteric function.

The Basic Function of the Sacred Trinity

The basic function of The Sacred Trinity of Radiant Health is to provide you with a greater understanding of the emotional, mental and physical bodies. In the following sections, you will explore each of the three bodies, their specific individual components and how their components operate. By grasping the basic workings of the three bodies, you can take charge of your physical, mental and emotional health and well-being. Radiant Health can only be experienced, however, when the Sacred Trinity's esoteric function is fulfilled.

The Esoteric Function of the Sacred Trinity

The esoteric function of the Sacred Trinity goes far beyond the study of the three individual bodies. Its higher purpose is to help you dissolve the illusion of who you think you are and provide you with information that can be put into action. Ultimately, action turns information into knowledge through experience. In this way you will come to understand your true nature: a Spirit that has taken human form. The design of the Sacred Trinity contains a formula to fulfill its esoteric role. The formula is to put the basic and exalted Spiritual qualities, contained in the center of each body, into action. Demonstrate them in your life and the ego characteristics (see Chapter 27) can be transcended. When the basic Spiritual component in the center of each of three bodies in the Sacred Trinity merges, integration occurs, and the ego, humanity's lower nature, is extinguished and the Spirit, humanity's higher nature, rises to the surface.

The Triangle Supports Synthesis and Integration

The triangle is the most stable structure known in the universe. When the three bodies are unified, synthesis is achieved, Spirit manifests, and the esoteric function of the Sacred Trinity is fulfilled. You are then connected by experiential realization to that which you are in reality. As a result of the Darkness, the natural balance between masculine and feminine energy has been disturbed. The Sacred Trinity's exalted purpose is to show you how to bring your masculine and feminine energies back into harmony. As you achieve your own "harmonic convergence," your Divine Child will spring to life. The Divine Child, when completely awakened, has a pure heart and lives fully present in the here and now. The Divine Child expresses the nature of Spirit in every moment.

The statement below is the foundation of step two on *The Journey to Radiant Health,* and combines the fundamental Spiritual qualities found in the center of each body of the Sacred Trinity. The statement comprises the Sacred Trinity's most simple yet most profound and powerful meaning. Applying its message to your life ensures integration of your three bodies and the experiential realization of Radiant Health:

Love is the highest *Truth* one can put into *Action*.

(Emotional)   *(Mental)*   *(Physical)*

This statement is a reminder that love is the most powerful Spiritual quality that defines us as human beings. The problem is that the Darkness of the Kali Yuga caused us to forget that we are Spiritual beings having a human experience. Instead we have been deluded into believing that we are human beings in search of a Spiritual experience. Therefore, the essential work on *The Journey to Radiant Health* is to recognize and correct this transposition. Then we can express the love that is the unlimited source of our power as Spiritual beings.

Love emits the highest frequency in the universe, and is the agent that binds everything together. Love binds the three bodies by way of the basic Spiritual qualities. Love is also exemplified in the exalted Spiritual qualities contained in each body's center. A chart of each body can be found at the start of Sections Four to Six. In the center of each circle above the basic Spiritual quality, you will find the body's exalted Spiritual quality:

In the Emotional body: *Agape is the exalted Spiritual ideal of Love.*

In the Mental body: *Wisdom is the exalted Spiritual ideal of Truth.*

In the Physical body: *Service is the exalted Spiritual ideal of Action.*

By putting even one of the exalted Spiritual qualities into action, the frequency of love can be transmitted through the other two bodies. Put love into action and it will dissolve any dissonant frequency. Even fear, which causes disharmony or dis-ease in the three bodies, will eventually disappear.

A wonderful window of opportunity exists during this process. It works like this: put the first and second steps on *The Journey to Radiant Health* into practice and anything of a lower vibration, including thoughts and emotions produced by fear, will rise to the surface. At that point, you can act to identify and dissolve these lower-nature, dissonant frequencies that keep you from living in the moment, enjoying your life and being of service to humanity.

The statement *"Love is the highest Truth one can put into Action"* also reminds you to look within and become grounded in Spirit before taking action. Introspection is key to obtaining Spiritual insight, revelation and direction. Making a consistent, conscious effort to integrate love and truth in every action will result in better relationships, stronger families and communities and a healthier world.

Combining, love, truth and action restores and maintains the balance and harmonic resonance of everything found in nature and the universe. As the frequency of love integrates the three bodies, you will experience emotional stability, mental clarity and physical vitality.

The Elements of the Sacred Trinity

The Sacred Trinity of Radiant Health, which has many layers and meanings, will be reviewed element by element. The three circles within the Sacred Trinity represent each of your three bodies. Each circle contains the individual components found within that particular body. The red circle at the top of the triangle represents the physical body. The yellow circle at the lower left of the triangle represents the mental body, and the blue circle at the lower right represents the emotional body.

Each of the three bodies contains a specific universal energy.

Mental body energy is masculine in nature. Among other spheres, masculine energy rules the right side of the body, logic, structure, discipline, thoughts, tolerance, will power, information, patience, organization, focus, truth and wisdom. Masculine energy moves in a linear direction and fixates itself on a specific point.

Emotional body energy is feminine in nature. Among other traits, feminine energy rules the heart, the left side of the body, love, creativity, tenderness, nurturing, kindness, experiences, forgiveness, compassion, acceptance, passion, emotions and Agape. Feminine energy moves in a circular direction and encompasses all things. Physical body energy represents the Divine Child. Balanced in its expression, the Divine Child is comprised of masculine and feminine energy. It rules the entire body and maintains its harmony. Free flowing and fluid in its expression, the Divine Child lives in awe of nature, honors life's mysteries and holds miracles as sacred. The Divine Child energy represents perfect equilibrium and harmony with innocent, inspirational, spontaneous and authentic qualities.

The Significance of the Sacred Trinity's Colors

The Sacred Trinity's colors signify relationships to the bodies. The emotional body's primary color is blue, which represents the fluidity of your emotions. When you align with Agape—the emotional body's exalted Spiritual quality—its primary color changes from blue to the rainbow spectrum. The rainbow reflects your ability to honor the similarities between you and others, respect the differences and live in the light of love. The mental body's primary color is yellow, which represents the process of mental assimilation. When you align with Wisdom—the mental body's exalted Spiritual quality—its primary color changes from yellow to gold. Gold reflects the strength of character required to hold oneself to the highest virtues, the standards of love and truth. The physical body's primary color is red, which represents action, and the integration of the masculine and feminine energy. When you align with Service—the physical body's exalted Spiritual quality—its primary color changes from red to clear. Clear emits all colors of the rainbow and enables you to clearly see others and yourself and vice versa, and know, intuitively, what to do to serve their needs.

The Outer Layers of the Sacred Trinity

The outermost layer in each of the three bodies contains three fundamental components. All nine components can be manipulated by the ego, which is part of the personality, or purified by the heart, which is part of Spirit. The fundamental components in each body are as follows:

The *Emotional body*:   Emotion, Experiences, Passion
The *Mental body*:   Thoughts, Information, Will
The *Physical body*:   Nourishment, Rest, Exercise

Historical Archetypes of Sacred Trinities

According to archaeologists, long before God was given the title Creator, Goddess held the position. Archaeological explorations of the most ancient civilizations, religions and cultures on Earth bear this out.

Artifacts such as small clay figures and sculptures point to the fact that the Matriarch was worshiped as the creator. Goddess artifacts have been unearthed at sites ranging from the Upper Paleolithic cultures dating back some 25,000 years, to the agricultural development that defined Neolithic communities[1]. In the Egyptian religion, the oldest known religion to humanity, the Goddess Isis is established in the feminine position as the prominent deity. In modern religions, the Patriarch is worshiped as the deity of creation. Modern civilizations and cultures are founded on the principle of the Patriarch as ruler. It is the masculine model that has been granted dominion over all.

The Matriarch had her day and the Patriarch is having his.

During the coming shift, the Matriarch and Patriarch will merge and give birth to the Divine Child—The Sacred Trinity of Radiant Health's model of supreme balance. The Sacred Trinity mirrors a host of religious, physical and metaphysical trinities that model perfect balance. For example, Christianity and Catholicism are founded on the Sacred Trinity of the God as the Father, Jesus as the Son and the Holy Ghost as the Spirit. In Hinduism, Brahma as the Creator, Vishnu as the Preserver and Shiva as the Dissolver reflect the Sacred Trinity. In the Egyptian religion the Sacred Trinity consists of Isis as the Mother, Osirus as the Father and Horus as the Son. The Kabbalah, the Judaic book of mysticism, has the Sacred Trinity as the upper three positions in the Tree of Life. Kethar (the Crown) represents the head, Binah (Understanding) the Primal Mother and Chokmah (Wisdom) the Father. The triangle creates perfect stability and every Sacred Trinity's stability—whether physical, religious or metaphysical—is created by the offspring of the merging masculine and feminine energy.

PHYSICAL AND METAPHYSICAL SYMBOLS
OF THE SACRED TRINITY

The Emotional Body	The Mental Body	The Physical Body
Mother/Feminine	Father/Masculine	Divine Child
Moon	Sun	Earth
Blue	Yellow	Red
Yin	Yang	Balance
Jing	Chi	Shen
Egg	Seed	Creation
Body	Mind	Spirit
Emotions	Thoughts	Sensations
Intuition	Instinct	Integration
Electron	Proton	Neutron
Moon sign	Rising sign	Sun sign
Meditation	Prayer	Dharma
Soul	Personality	Spirit
Who you think you are	Who others think you are	Who you really are
Future	Past	Present

Metaphysical Symbols Explained

Metaphysical Sacred Trinities also can be used to further your self-understanding. For example, take the Sacred Trinity of astrological signs: sun, rising and moon. The moon sign represents your feminine energy—who you think you are. It governs your emotions, needs, moods and how you care for and nurture others. The rising sign represents your masculine energy—who others think you are. It governs the ego/personality. The sun sign, designated by your birth date, represents the Divine Child—your true self. This is who you become when your masculine and feminine energies are integrated. Your astrological composition can be an invaluable tool to help you identify the ego, and understand how and what to change.

The body/mind/Spirit paradigm is another well-known Sacred Trinity. In this paradigm, the body represents the basic element of physical existence. The body can be mastered by the second element, the mind. Spirit, the final component in the paradigm, is the purest aspect of this Sacred Trinity. Unaffected by the laws of matter, Spirit resides beyond the mind and body and transcends the laws of physical reality. The mastery of Spirit results in omnipotence, omniscience and omnipresence, and has been achieved by notable Spiritual figures including Jesus of Nazareth, Buddha, Krisna, Mohammed and Lao Tze.

The Sacred Trinity of Prayer, Meditation and Dharma

Steps two and three on *The Journey to Radiant Health* are comprised of the most important and powerful Sacred Trinity: Prayer, Meditation and Dharma—right action. Prayer is the act of making a petition or declaration to Spirit. Meditation is the act of sitting in silence, and turning one's focus and attention inward to receive an answer to the prayer. Both are key Spiritual components in seeking and connecting with the Divine. Dharma is the conscious, loving application of the direction you receive through your prayer and meditation. The application of this Sacred Trinity ensures that you are divinely guided in all actions.

The Masculine Component: Prayer

Prayer is the most effective means for establishing direct contact with Spirit. Prayer brings you into direct alignment with Spirit externally, God, and internally, the heart. It enables you to gain clarity, especially when confusion or uncertainty arises. A clearly stated prayer, to seek direction or guidance, ask for help or find a solution to a problem, opens the mind and focuses it on a single point of thought. To enhance a prayer's effectiveness, it is imperative to recite the petition for a time period long enough to saturate the mind, which then dispatches a more magnified mental energy to Spirit. More information concerning this process can be found in "Affirmations, Bhajans, and Mantras," Chapter 21. Prayer is the most effective means to keep the mind aligned and focused on Spirit, and minimize or banish the Darkness and its most destructive qualities, fear, greed, anger, lust, hatred and laziness.

PRAYER EXERCISE

1. Choose a Master, Angel, Saint, Enlightened Being or God Itself. Examples; Jesus, Buddha, Quan Yin, Mother Mary, Allah, Jehovah, Saint Germaine, Archangel Michael, Krishna, Ganesh, Subramanya, Hanuman, etc.

2. Each morning when you wake up, pray to your chosen Deity to embody its Love, and be guided in your actions and protected from harm.

3. Each evening, before you go to sleep, send a prayer of thanks for embodying its Love and being guided in your actions and protected from harm.

The Feminine Component: Meditation

Meditation is the balancing component to prayer. After a specific prayer has been enacted, then one sits in silence in order to obtain direction, guidance or an answer to the prayer. This is one form of meditation. Each of the conscious breathing exercises outlined in Chapters 4 and 7 can also be used as a focus for meditation. Meditation, the feminine activity of opening the heart to receive, enables you to commune with Spirit and draw wisdom from higher conscious beings. Meditation is the cornerstone to procure information, direction and guidance on how to put love into action. Throughout *The Journey to Radiant Health* you will find a number of meditation exercises that will help open your heart and make your journey successful.

MEDITATION EXERCISE

1. Place a picture of your chosen Deity in the area that you do your conscious breathing practice.

2. Sit quietly and gaze at the picture for a few minutes.

3. Close your eyes, focus on your breath and open your heart.

4. For the next ten minutes, try to feel the Divine energy and Love and presence of your chosen Deity.

Use Prayer and Meditation to Find Your Dharma

Dharma is defined as "right conduct, right action and right liveli-hood." Pursue your Dharma and you contribute to the well-being of others and welfare of your community. On *The Journey to Radiant Health,* conscious breathing is the discipline that enables you to quiet the mind, open the heart, find your Dharma and put it into action. Conscious breathing prepares you to pray with single-minded clarity and meditate with open-hearted receptivity. When abstract thoughts are minimized and the heart is fully open, you can receive clear information, direction and guidance from your angels, guides and Spirit. Prayer and meditation will help you ascertain your Dharma. Formulate a clear intentioned prayer and send it to your chosen Deity. Ask that your Dharma be revealed. When the prayer has saturated your mind, meditate to open your heart and receive the information about your Dharma. If no answer comes, do not fret. In Chapter 17 you will have the opportunity to meet your Spirit Child. Your Spirit Child holds the key to your Dharma and will guide you to it.

Conscious Breathing Integrates the Three Bodies

Conscious breathing can be the single most effective tool to inte-grate the three bodies and facilitate Radiant Health. Conscious breathing brings a greater supply of oxygen to the blood, removes more carbon dioxide and other toxins and increases your overall physical energy. It quiets the mind and enables you to develop greater mental focus and concentration. It also keeps your creative emotional energy flowing freely.

Apply step one on *The Journey to Radiant Health,* and as conscious breathing becomes the foundation for your life, your awareness will grow, and in time and with practice, integration of the three bodies will occur. Apply step two, the Sacred Trinity's most powerful tenet—Love is the highest Truth that one can put into Action—and with the help of step three, this Spiritual statement can become the conscious focus for everything you do.

9

Duality Within
the Sacred Trinity

For thousands of years, Oriental and Ayervedic medicine and other healing arts have applied the principles of Yin and Yang to the human body to restore balance. Yin and Yang define the laws of duality. By examining the underlying principles of Yin and Yang, the duality found in everything in nature can be understood, and then transcended to reach the higher ground of Spirit.

The physical body in and of itself, and the emotional and mental bodies together, symbolize your descent from wholeness into the dualistic state of opposites. To overcome the limitations of duality, it is essential to recognize, accept and harmonize your masculine- and feminine-based qualities. When the emotional and mental bodies are integrated, you will recognize and transcend duality, and the ego perception of being separate and different from others will dissolve.

In The Sacred Trinity of Radiant Health, the Divine Child symbolizes the transcendence of duality and a return to your inherent state of Divine perfection. The Divine Child expresses the feminine Spirit quality, love, in balance with its masculine Spirit quality counterpart, truth. As the pure Spirit state of Oneness is re-established, you will live in peace and harmony with all things.

Yin and Yang: The Balance of Opposites

The term *Yin* describes the principle of feminine/receptive energy, while *Yang* describes the principle of masculine/active energy. The elements of Yin and Yang constitute the whole of everything in physical existence. According to the principle of Yin and Yang, everything that exists in nature manifests in pairs and is governed by cycles. As one element advances its partner/opposite recedes, and while the energy of one partner is always dominant, the energy of the other is always present.

Yin and Yang co-exist within the whole as they continually ebb and flow in a state of perfect harmonious opposites. In the physical body, as in nature, when the energy in one pathway stagnates or is blocked, the natural rhythm is disrupted and both are thrown out of balance. The restoration of energy to its natural rhythm and flow ensures the return of balance and the recovery of health and well-being.

The following page contains the ancient Yin/Yang symbol. The "S" shaped line that divides Yin from Yang, and yet connects them, is a symbolic representation of the idea of the *middle path*—that which is beyond duality. The *middle path*, the foundation of the Buddha's teachings, is a formula for transcending duality. The black symbol represents the Yin element, the white symbol represents the Yang element. The black dot within the white symbol, and vice versa, indicates that one always exists within the other.

On the following page are some examples of Yin and Yang as they exist in the balanced dance of opposites. The verse from the Nei Jing reflects universal truth as it pertains to duality.

Although duality is a valid expression of the physical world, it is born of Maya—the illusion produced by Darkness. To transcend duality, synthesize your masculine and feminine energy and experience Radiant Health, it is necessary to raise your frequency and your awareness. The conscious breathing exercises in Section Two, along with the meditation practices contained in *The Journey to Radiant Health,* enable you to do this by opening your heart, connecting with Spirit and experiencing its Light.

The Buddha also left humanity with a simple and effective formula for transcending duality. The Spiritual discipline known as "Vipassana" is the practice the Buddha prescribed for achieving enlightenment. The Annapana technique—your first conscious breathing

YIN		YANG
Cold		Hot
Female		Male
Left		Right
Wet		Dry
Night		Day
Slow		Fast
Soft		Hard
Moon		Sun
Internal		External
Winter		Summer
Receptive		Active
Dark		Light

Yin has its root in Yang
Yang has its root in Yin
Without Yin, Yang cannot arise
Without Yang, Yin cannot be born
Yin alone cannot arise; Yang alone cannot grow
Yin and Yang are divisible but inseparable

—Nei Jing

exercise—precedes the practice of Vipassana. Annapana distills the mind and develops focus and concentration. A Vipassana course[1] teaches one to transcend the duality found in the physical world. The practice enables one to walk "the middle path," detach from sense objects and thus avoid life's highs and lows.

This is the foundation of the Buddha's teachings.

The physical body is the Divine Temple and yet within it resides the Spirit. In the Body/Mind/Spirit Trinity, the focus is to recognize and move beyond the Maya of Darkness that hides your Spirit and causes you to believe that you are the body. Put the seven *Journey to Radiant Health* steps into action and you will uncover and come into direct contact with your Spirit.

Which Is Your Primary Body?

To achieve balance, the first step is to identify the primary body from which you act: emotional or mental. After identifying the primary body, you can consciously work to strengthen your use of the components in the opposite body. The emotional and mental bodies are like muscles; without stimulation they atrophy. In accordance with the principle of Yin and Yang, one is usually dominant. Finding your primary body and then exercising and strengthening your use of the components in the opposite body is an effective way to develop the balance needed to walk the "middle path."

The following questions will clarify whether your actions tend to lean more towards the emotional or mental body. Circle your answer to each question.

1. Which are you more apt to follow?   *Emotions* or *Thoughts*

2. Which do you rely on when making decisions?   *Information* or *Experiences*

3. What drives you to your goals?   *Will* or *Passion*

The basic emotional body components are Emotions, Experiences and Passion. The basic mental body components are Thoughts, Information and Will Power. Which body received the majority of your answers, emotional or mental? Your answers can help determine which body needs to be strengthened in order for you to achieve balance. If all three of your answers came from the emotional body, then the mental body needs to be strengthened. If the opposite is true, then the emotional body needs to be strengthened. If two of your answers came from the mental body and one from the emotional body, or vice versa, then you are already on your way towards balance. Work to strengthen the opposite body and you will integrate the two and achieve balance.

Human beings express duality in a multitude of ways. The duality between thoughts and emotions, information and experiences, and will and passion are just a few examples. The metaphysical symbols of human duality—woman and man—play an essential part in the process of conception. A woman provides the egg and a man provides the seed. As the pair comes together, duality falls away and a whole new life is brought forth.

The Disintegrative Effects
of the Ego

There is one element in the human make-up that can keep you from experiencing Radiant Health. Master this element, and you will experience peace of mind, connection with your Spirit, love for all things and Radiant Health.

The element is the ego.

The mental body houses the ego and an in-depth discussion pertaining to it can be found in the mental body section (Section Five). In The Sacred Trinity of Radiant Health, every outer layer component in each of the three bodies is susceptible to the ego's influence. This chapter outlines how the ego blocks the Sacred Trinity's natural pathway and flow of energy between the three bodies. Also outlined are the basic dis-eases that take place in each body when the flow of energy between them is disrupted by the ego.

How Energy Flows through the Three Bodies

Energy descends from the Spirit realm and enters the emotional body. The emotional body carries the Spirit egg of love, whose energy provides Divine inspiration, visions, dreams and imagination. The feminine/emotional body passes its egg into the masculine/mental body, where the seed of truth is added, whose energy provides structure, organization and alignment with the Divine. The impregnated energy then passes into the physical body where it is birthed into physical reality as action, or Dharma, completing the cycle. When energy follows this route through the three bodies, your creative potential can be fully expressed and you can experience Radiant Health.

But the ego can disrupt the process.

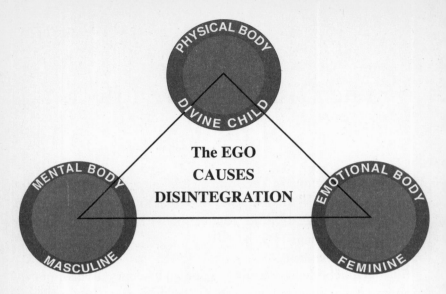

The Disintegrative Effects of the Ego

Disintegration occurs when fear arises and the ego is allowed to deny or suppress the fear. In effect, the ego severs the energetic cord that connects the emotional, mental and physical bodies, causing them to appear separate from one another. Sever the natural connection between the three bodies, and the release of fear becomes impossible and dis-ease is likely to occur.

If dis-ease is not experienced immediately, it will manifest at some later point in time. When the ego is allowed to prevent the emotional body's energy from following its natural pathway, the energy is internalized. Energy, however, does not stop flowing. When a natural pathway is blocked, the energy continues to build. Energy, being a fluid medium, will eventually find an alternative outlet. The end result is disintegration; and the displaced energy manifests as an emotional, mental or physical dis-ease.

The ego is always at the root of disintegration.

The healthy way to express fear is to allow its energy to follow its natural pathway through the three bodies. First, the emotional body *feels it*. Next, the mental body *identifies and acknowledges* the fear, which includes the cover-feelings, anger or sadness. Finally, the physical body can *release the energy* of the fear through conscious breathing.

Listed below are the core effects of disintegration. The effects are specific to each individual body.

When the ego blocks your mental body energy,
only the emotional and physical body energies are active,
and the basic effect is:

Blind Love

Without the balance of truth, reason and wisdom are destroyed
and destructive behaviors like co-dependency, enabling
and addictions take hold.

When the ego blocks your emotional body energy,
only the physical and mental body energies are active,
and the basic effect is:

Truth Destroys

Spoken without the balance of compassion,
the sharp blades of truth cut the recipient to shreds.
Rather than healing, it opens a bleeding wound.

When the ego blocks your physical body energy,
only the mental and emotional body energies are active,
and the basic effect is:

Procrastination

The energy needed to turn imagination and dreams into
physical reality is absent, and laziness replaces activity.

The Four Pathways of Energy

As energy passes through the emotional body it takes one of four different routes. Three of the pathways are unhealthy, and are rooted in the ego and cause disintegration. The healthy pathway is rooted in the heart, is the unlimited source of your Divine power and Spiritual potential and leads to Radiant Health. It will be covered in the beginning of the next chapter.

The three unhealthy outlets are accidents, reactions and dis-ease.

Accidents

What are defined as accidents are not accidents at all. Accidents happen when your focus and attention has been distracted from the immediate task at hand. The distraction is created by an emotion that was not identified, acknowledged and expressed at the moment it was experienced. As a result, instead of paying attention to what you are doing, your energy is wrapped up in thinking about how you feel about what was said, what you wished you would have said or what you wished would have happened. Being distracted from the task at hand such as walking, cutting vegetables or driving a car results in physical injuries such as sliced fingers, broken limbs or even possibly death.

Reactions

Reactions are a result of fear and occur when an incident opens an unhealed wound, which triggers a spontaneous, volcanic emotional explosion. Emotional energy and its effects will be discussed in detail in the next section. Suffice to say here that the emotional energy produced by reactions can be just as harmful or deadly as an accident. Reactions can cause harsh words to be spoken, property to be destroyed or violence perpetrated. In extreme cases it can result in murder or suicide. Reactions can be overcome by the use of conscious breathing. Also, on page 95 and throughout Section Four, you will find exercises that will enable you to harness destructive emotional energy and shift it to constructive energy.

Dis-ease

Dis-ease will be covered thoroughly in the following three sections. For now, know that the repression of emotional energy leads to dis-ease. Repressing emotions stifles creative energy and stops the pursuit of your dreams. Repressing emotions also results from the fear of experiencing the intense emotions of painful or traumatic experiences. Denying the emotions locks them deep into the recesses of the mind. In each case, the creative/emotional energy is not given an outlet. Rather than being released it stews in the mind, often for many years. The consequences that arise from this blocked emotional energy are severe and can also be deadly. After a period of time, the long-standing, unresolved and unexpressed emotional conflict will materialize as a major, or deadly, physical dis-ease such as heart disease or cancer. It can also manifest in emotional and mental dis-eases including breakdowns, depression and obsessions.

Use the Sacred Trinity As a Paradigm for Living

Practice conscious breathing and follow the Sacred Trinity's simple script—*Love is the highest Truth one can put into Action*—and you have a simple paradigm for living. These two steps will cause your awareness to grow by leaps and bounds and enable you to experience a life of unending joy and Radiant Health. But the Sacred Trinity can take you even further.

Living Your Life As a Divine Child

The Divine Child is positioned at the top of the Sacred Trinity precisely because its energy transcends duality. The Divine Child integrates and harmonizes masculine and feminine energy, enabling you to recognize and ascend beyond limiting ideas and belief systems—ideas and beliefs that, founded in duality, cause you to feel separate from others because of external differences like gender, race, color, religion, heritage and class.

Live in the heart and become the Divine Child that rises to meet its Spirit. The top of the triangle represents the experience of interconnectedness and unity with all things. The Divine Child exemplifies peace of mind and fairness of heart. This makes it possible for you to simultaneously express love and truth in all interactions.

The Divine Child represents the pure Spirit that exists in you. Free from regrets of the past or worries about the future, the Divine Child experiences every moment in the perfectly awakened state of conscious awareness. When you awaken the Divine Child within, you will experience each moment as a new beginning. You will experience life with wonder and awe for the miracles that most people take for granted: daily miracles like waking to a new day, smelling a fragrant flower, viewing a sunrise or sunset, or meeting someone for the first or the hundredth time.

Your life will take on a whole new perspective.

Learn to see Spirit in everything and you will take nothing for granted. You will not cling to the past, but will fully trust that everything is divinely orchestrated and is always in perfect order. Best of all, as you embody the wholeness of the Divine Child you will be liberated from the Maya of separation, loneliness and suffering.

A Final Note on Duality.

No exploration of duality would be complete without exploring its most fundamental manifestations: love and fear. Love and fear are the only two active forces in the universe and every action, whether conscious or not, stems from one or the other.

Fear is a contractive energy.

Love is an expansive energy.

Love and fear are never acted out simultaneously. To experience Radiant Health, it is imperative to act from love, while recognizing and acknowledging fear. Each energy will be explored in great detail throughout the book.

SECTION FOUR

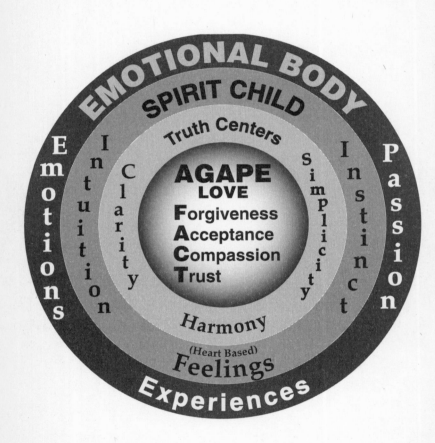

Color chart available at:
www.radiantkeys.com

The Emotional Body

Start the day with love,
Fill the day with love,
Spend the day with love,
End the day with love.
This is the way to God.

—Sai Baba

The three bodies of the Sacred Trinity are akin to seeds. Each body needs proper nurturing and attention to sprout, grow strong and remain healthy. Proper nurturing and attention means learning how each body operates and using what is learned to keep their energy flowing freely. When energy flows unencumbered through each body, you will experience Radiant Health.

Although the emotional and mental bodies are balancing partners and equal in their energetic importance, the emotional body comes first because feminine energy gives birth to all things in creation, regardless of whether it is negative or positive, destructive or constructive, limited or unlimited. The feminine energy of the emotional body is housed in the heart and symbolized by the circle. The heart governs all relationships, and holds each one in a light of sacred reverence. The heart is quiet, calm and steady; it does not worry, judge or panic. It moves to the natural rhythm of life. The heart enjoys, accepts, forgives, embraces, supports and, most of all, it trusts.

While the mind needs to figure things out, the heart trusts
that whatever needs to be known will be revealed.

The Healthy Energy Pathway

In the previous chapter you learned that only one healthy pathway exists for the expression of your emotional body's energy. This outlet is the Radiant key that keeps the emotional body's energy flowing consistently, even during the most challenging moments of your life.

The healthy outlet is unconditional love: Agape.

Agape is creative energy. An open heart keeps you connected to Spirit, and a never-ending flow of Agape's creative energy pours from the loving heart of a healthy emotional body. Creative loving expression is key for you to experience lasting peace, serenity and happiness. To experience Radiant Health, it is essential for you to open your heart and put Agape's creative energy to work.

An infinite number of possibilities for creative expression can be imagined and explored. Your creative potential is fettered only by the mind's inability to comprehend the reality of infinity. Learning to listen to your heart and act on its messages is the best method for actualizing your heart's creative potential. The heart is the connection to your empathic, sensitive nature. It is a vessel of light that enables you to see beyond the darkness, transcend the illusion of duality, align with Spirit and put love into action.

The heart can heal all wounds and dispel all fears.

The heart is home to love-based qualities such as forgiveness, acceptance, compassion, trust, gentleness, kindness, devotion and, most of all, love. Heart-based qualities flow freely from a healthy emotional body. An open heart enables you to receive and give love and serve others. Healthy families, communities and relationships are cultivated and sustained by putting the full list of the heart's qualities (found in Chapter 19) into practice.

The Outer Layer of the Emotional Body: Emotions, Passion and Experiences

The first step toward actualizing radiant emotional health is to identify and release from the emotional body that which does not support the vibration of love—specifically, the ego-based emotions, perceptions, attitudes and belief systems that cause you to react rather than respond to your environment.

Reactions arise from the ego/fear.

Responses arise from the heart/love.

At the core of any fear-based ego belief are the experiences, emotions and passions that have been judged as negative, bad or harmful. Judgments are caused by reactions and do not support the vibration of love. Judging any emotions, experiences or passions negates your ability to embody and act from love. When the mental body's constructive components—focus, discipline and commitment—are used in alliance with the emotional body's truth centers—instinct, intuition and heart-based feelings—the ego's behaviors, including judgment, are exposed and can be eliminated.

In Section Five you will learn how to use the constructive components and the truth centers for this purpose. In the meantime, you can get a head start by learning how to identify and release the judgments of experiences, emotions and passions that cause you to suffer.

Emotions

Emotions are energy, and every emotion you feel is totally and completely valid. However, what you choose to do with the energy of your emotions is the most powerful determining factor in whether you will experience Radiant Health or dis-ease. As you discovered in Section 3, denied or repressed emotions will eventually find an outlet that produces dis-ease. To experience Radiant Health, emotional energy needs to be managed and expressed in a proactive way. As an equation, emotions can be written as:

"E-motion = energy in motion"

The equation suggests that emotional energy is always in motion. Without structure, the emotional body's creative energy turns chaotic.

Feel, Identify and Own Your Emotions

Judging emotions is a major obstacle on *The Journey to Radiant Health*. Intuitively, fear-based emotions are recognized as being unhealthy, but judging them leads to repression, denial or more destructive explosive forms of behavior like hatred, violence or suicide. Initially, denied or repressed emotions simply block your creative energy. When they remain buried inside you, they eventually lead to acute or chronic emotional, mental and/or physical dis-ease. Conscious breathing enables you to feel your emotions. This first step on the Journey to Radiant Emotional Health leads directly to the next step, being able to identify emotions. After you have identified the emotions, the next step is to take ownership and responsibility for the way they make you feel. This empowers you to do something healthy with them. If you do not own your emotions, you will instead blame others for how you feel. For example, you might say, *"You are making me angry. If you would just be nice, I would be happy."*

No one has the power to make you feel any emotion.

You have the power of choice to determine whether you react or respond. By choosing to respond to the emotions you feel, you can own and express them in ways that do not harm others.

Analyzing Emotions Leads to Avoidance

A common way to avoid experiencing emotions in the moment is by trying to figure out what caused them. This occurs when conscious breathing is not implemented and the ego is allowed to react to a feeling. This is a major contributing factor in the cause of emotional, mental and eventually physical dis-ease.

Do not analyze your emotions.

To keep your emotional energy flowing freely, apply this Radiant Key: feel your emotions as they arise. Do not stop to analyze them. Stopping to analyze your emotions is the ego's way to trick you into thinking your way out of experiencing what you are feeling. Sometimes emotions cause discomfort. It's not fun to feel sad or angry, but thinking about your emotions, rather than feeling them, blocks the flow of your emotional body's creative energy.

Because a host of external factors can influence how you feel, analyzing your emotions is futile. For example, the moon's gravitational pull exerts tremendous pressure on every body of water in the world. Your body, which is composed of up to 80% water, is also subject to the moon's gravitational force. During the full portion of the lunar cycle, the moon's gravitational pressure gives rise to intensified feelings and emotions. It is well documented that episodes of confrontation, violence and other emotional outbursts escalate during the days around a full moon cycle.

Analysis cannot stop or change this phenomenon.

Because your emotional state can be affected by factors beyond your control, understanding how you feel will not always change how you feel. This is why conscious breathing is critical to your health and well-being. Conscious breathing brings awareness to what you are feeling without reaction. Awareness enables you to experience a wide variety of emotional, mental or physical pressures without reacting to them.

Masking Emotions

"Masks" are used to hide emotions. Historically, boys have worn "masks" to disguise or deny the empathic side of their nature. This includes repressing their more sensitive and tender emotions. Should a boy cry, be close to his mother or exhibit any feminine-based emotions or traits, he runs the risk of being insulted or tagged with disparaging labels such as sissy, faggot or wimp. Even worse, he could become the target of violence.

Disparaging labels or attacks can leave deep scars.

Messages like *"be a man," "boys don't cry"* or *"suck it up"* can adversely affect a boy's self-confidence and damage his overall emotional health and well-being. Because crying is more acceptable for a girl and anger is not, she is likely to mask emotions when she feels angry. Messages like *"girls are not leaders," "it is not lady-like to be angry," "girls are weak"* or *"it's a man's world"* are detrimental to her emotional health and well-being. Messages like these can undermine her self-confidence, as well as her aspirations to set and achieve exalted goals.

Men can have a powerful and healthy impact on children by displaying their own tender, heart-felt emotions. This will teach children, especially boys, that it is okay to feel and share them. Women can have a powerful and healthy impact on children by constructively channeling their anger and displaying strength and decisiveness in their actions. This will teach children, especially girls, that everyone can lead. This basic recipe for modeling emotions in a healthy way will help boys and girls grow into healthy and emotionally mature men and women.

Modeling Radiant Emotional Health for Children

Raising an emotionally healthy child predominantly depends on parents and caregivers to model emotionally healthy behaviors. This means it is necessary to evaluate your own emotional health. Be bold; explore your own belief systems, behaviors and actions—because children imitate what they see much more than listening to what they are told.

How you act is most often a direct result of what you witnessed and experienced in your home. What you were taught overtly and what you learned covertly are not always the same thing. The adage *"Do as I say, not as I do"* does not work. Children learn by watching and imitating actions. This is known as modeling. You have the power to model healthy emotional behavior by healing the wounds that have contributed to your unhealthy behaviors.

If you were conditioned to believe any of the previous messages, or your beliefs, behaviors or actions are not based in love, examine your experiences. Childhood is the best place to start, and in Chapter 17 you will meet your Spirit Child and have an opportunity to uncover and examine those experiences. Then you can re-evaluate your belief systems, perceptions and attitudes. You can also make changes to ensure that you do not hand down unhealthy behavior patterns to your children.

Radiant Health in Interpersonal Relationships

Radiant Health in relationships depends on awareness and taking responsibility for your emotions. This means being able to feel, identify, own and ultimately change the emotions that lead to reactive emotional displays such as yelling, blaming or being critical or judgmental.

It is not necessary to be perfect.

It is necessary to make a decision to do the work that leads to change. When your emotions are intense, begin conscious breathing. If the intensity of the emotions is overwhelming, find a healthy physical outlet to dissipate the energy. For example, go for a walk or run, or pound pillows with a tennis racket, or put on protective gloves and hit a punching bag. When the content of the emotional energy subsides, your feelings can be expressed without personalizing, judging, blaming or engaging in other unhealthy behaviors. If you find that you are still too agitated to communicate your feelings, then remain silent and continue to practice conscious breathing until the energy subsides. Below are three basic rules for keeping yourself and others safe while expressing the energy of emotions.

1. *Do not harm yourself.*
2. *Do not harm anyone else.*
3. *Do not destroy property.*

When emotions are withheld, denied or repressed, the opportunity to experience what you are feeling in the moment is lost, never to be felt again in that particular way. In other words, when feelings are denied, you lose the opportunity to feel what you are feeling in the moment. Although you might be able to return (in your mind) to that moment, the purity of emotion in that moment has been lost. The opportunity to overcome the resistance to feeling the uncomfortable emotions, or judgments about the emotions, has been lost as well. Further, when emotions are denied expression, the energy is deposited in some region of the physical body's cellular structure. For example, if you feel angry and clench your jaw rather than express the anger, then the emotional energy becomes lodged in the jaw. The anger energy will remain in the jaw until it is identified, owned, expressed and released, or until it manifests as a physical dis-ease—such as TMJ, teeth grinding or interrupted sleep. When a physical, emotional or mental dis-ease manifests, it can be a red flag alerting you to uncover repressed or denied emotions.

Bodywork, rebirthing, acupressure, cranial sacral therapy and other forms of energy and breath work are powerful tools that assist the healing process. Energy work helps to expose and clear blocked emotional energy, and alleviate stress, tension and dis-ease from the physical body. Energy work also restores your creative energy, which reestablishes Radiant Health. As a by-product of working to heal, you will also experience healthier relationships. The adage *better late than never* always applies when you are working to release past emotions.

Confusion

Fear is the root of all dis-ease-producing emotions. One of the most destructive emotions fear produces is confusion. Co-dependent behavior arises from fear, and is characterized by denying or repressing your own emotions in order to keep others happy. Fear causes you to avoid the discomfort of expressing your true feelings, which in turn produces internal conflict, which in turn leads to confusion. When the ego projects fears of what others will think of you, or how they will react if you express your feelings, co-dependent behavior and emotional withholding are inevitable.

Fear-based thoughts that lead to co-dependent behavior include: *"If I tell him that I am angry, he will attack me," "If she knows how I feel, she will reject me," "I feel sad, but if I cry, they will think that I am weak" or "I feel angry, but if I tell her, she will think I am mean or insensitive."* The underlying fear causes the ego to create a conflict between what you think and how you feel. Your feelings are valid but the ego, fearing what others might think or say if you express your feelings, causes you to withhold or invalidate them.

> *The only time confusion arises is when the ego represses your heart's natural feelings.*

To eliminate confusion, return the mind's focus to conscious breathing, and feel what you are feeling. Open your heart and own your emotions and you will be able to express them in a responsible healthy way. Keep in mind that 99% of the time the first feeling that arises comes from the heart, and that 99% of the time the first thought that arises comes from ego.

Repressing or denying emotions stifles your creative, feeling aspect, and also robs others of an opportunity to learn and grow; sharing your feelings gives others an opportunity to learn about you. Healthy relationships are created by being honest about how you feel, and expressing your emotions responsibly.

In the beginning, expressing your feelings might be awkward and uncomfortable, but you can work through the discomfort. The key is to practice. In time, it will become easier to express your emotions.

EXERCISE:
CLIMBING THE EMOTIONAL LADDER
TO RADIANT HEALTH

The emotional ladder to Radiant Health will guide you to healthy emotional expression. Climb it and you will feel a new sense of empowerment.

Step 1. Feel Your Emotions.

When emotions arise, do not deny, repress or withhold them.

Turn your attention inward and feel the emotions' accompanying sensations—heat, pulsing, increased heart-beat.

Practice conscious breathing exercise #2.

Breathe into the sensations until their energy dissipates.

Step 2. Identify Your Emotions.

Continue to practice conscious breathing exercise #2. Identify the emotions—fear, anger or sadness—as they rise to the surface. Do not give up. It might take some time to identify the emotions. Be patient and stay with the process.

Step 3. Own Your Emotions.

Take responsibility for the emotions you are feeling.

Do not blame others for how you feel.

Do your best not to react to what has been said to you, how others are acting toward you or not getting what you want from a situation. Instead, continue to practice conscious breathing exercise #2.

Step 4. Express Your Emotions.

Remain silent until the emotions' sensations and energy have passed.

When you feel calm and centered, express the emotions in a healthy manner. Use "I" statements such as "I felt angry," "I felt hurt" or "I felt irritated."

If the emotion rises again, stop talking and return to conscious breathing exercise #2.

The greatest challenge with emotions is to ride the wave of feelings without reacting. Remember to remain silent until the energy subsides. Climb each step of the emotional ladder with honesty, integrity and an open heart. Do not allow the ego to remain in control, otherwise you will believe that you have climbed the ladder when you have not. Instead, you will have avoided feeling the feelings. Typically, this occurs when a principle is understood intellectually but has not been put it into practice. For example, reading a book on plumbing does not make one a plumber. The ego is a master of intellectualizing rather than practicing. The ego will try to remain in control, and will deny or repress your emotions as it attempts to create the appearance of being emotionally healthy.

Detachment Can Help You Achieve Emotional Mastery

When you have mastered the four steps on the emotional ladder of Radiant Health, you can begin to practice the Spiritual discipline of detachment. The purpose behind the Spiritual discipline of detachment is to achieve self-realization: the knowledge of your true self. Detachment will also help you achieve emotional mastery.

This is key to experiencing Radiant Health.

The first step in the Spiritual discipline of detachment is to identify the things to which you are attached. Attachments include a variety of things such as belief systems, desires or habits. You can also be attached to material things such as people, money, fame, beauty, power and sex. Ego behaviors such as selfishness, pride, lust, greed, envy and judgment are attachments. You can also be attached to a baseball team, a cause or the home in which you live or other objects.

The ego attaches to everything.

Attachments cause you to lose the perspective that everything existing in the world is temporary, in motion and subject to change. Loss of this perspective also leads to loss of objectivity, mental clarity and emotional centeredness.

Attachments are the root cause of suffering.

Detachment is a process by which you make a conscious decision to surrender your personal desires and attachments. It is a conscious letting go of the self-centered ego personality. Practice the Spiritual discipline of detachment consciously and consistently, and it will free you from anything to which you are attached.

But beware; the ego can make detachment difficult.

The ego personality has no desire to let go of control or surrender desires. Denial enables the ego personality to rationalize or justify selfish actions. The ego can also cause you to believe that because you intellectually understand the Spiritual discipline of detachment, you can by-pass expressing your emotions by claiming to be detached. Detachment is not a vehicle to deny your feelings.

The Spiritual discipline and practice of detachment is an open-hearted practice of awareness. Detachment exercises can be found in Chapters 21 and 27. The practice will enable you to gain a broader perspective on the true meaning of life. It will help you give all things equal consideration when making important decisions. Detachment helps you balance being firm and decisive with being considerate and compassionate.

This becomes possible because Spirit attaches to nothing.

Detachment leads to greater awareness and enables you to connect easily to Spirit. Being detached liberates you from suffering, and enables you to be objective, peaceful, centered and single-mindedly focused on Spirit, even in the midst of life's trials and tribulations. By mastering the practice of detachment, you will achieve self-realization and experience Radiant Health.

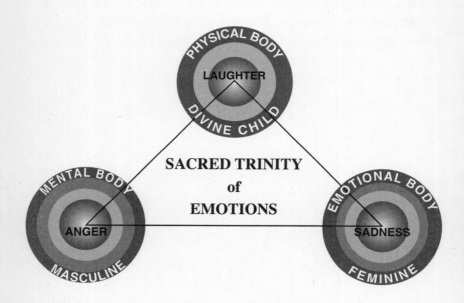

12

The Sacred Trinity of Anger, Sadness and

Although the emotions that can be experien~~ced~~ ~~are~~ ~~~~ ited, the entire spectrum can be traced to one of three emotions. They represent The Sacred Trinity of Emotions.

The three emotions are: Anger, Sadness and Laughter.

In The Sacred Trinity of Emotions, anger corresponds to mental body/masculine energy, sadness to the emotional body/feminine energy and laughter to the physical body/Divine Child energy. As discussed earlier, there are only two energies present in dualistic creation, fear and love. The root of anger and sadness is fear, while the root of laughter is love.

The Yin and Yang Emotions: Sadness and Anger

Sadness and anger exist on opposite ends of the emotional energy spectrum. Anger's energy is Yang, while sadness's energy is Yin. Both anger and sadness can be expressed by a wide range of unhealthy emotions. They vary in degrees of intensity and all produce dis-ease. When their energy is channeled into the heart, however, anger and sadness can promote health and well-being.

Awareness is the Radiant Key that enables you to harness and transform the destructive potential of anger and sadness into constructive health-promoting energies. Because the underlying energy of anger and sadness arises from fear, it is inherently destructive. When felt and identified, however, the energy can be shifted. The emotional energy of anger and sadness can be managed and then transformed by the practice of conscious breathing. Shift the emotional energy of anger and sadness from fear to love and the root energy changes from destructive to creative.

ANGER: THE MASCULINE EMOTION

Anger can be the most volatile, explosive and destructive of all emotions. Uncontrolled anger possesses the greatest threat to humanity and all sentient beings. Its divisive energy tears apart families, communities, nations and is a very real threat to all inhabitants of the world. The effects of uncontrolled anger are portrayed daily in mainstream media outlets such as TV, radio and newspapers, and are often the source of headline stories.

Uncontrolled anger will take you out of alignment with your Divine nature faster than anything else. But, the energy produced by anger is not strictly bad or negative. Anger's energy can be harnessed, channeled and transformed into creative expressions.

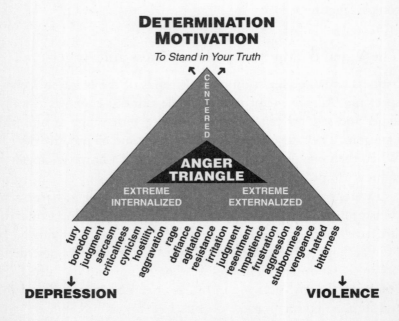

This section contains techniques that can help you transmute anger's energy from unhealthy, reactive and destructive to healthy, proactive and constructive. Because while others are liable to feel the effects of your anger, in the end it is you who experiences the lion's share of its dis-ease-producing energy. Before going further into the causes and effects of anger, take a moment and look at the anger triangle.

The Anger Triangle Explained

At the base of the anger triangle are its extreme polarities of unhealthy expression. Anger's most Yin/internalized expression is depression, while its most Yang/externalized expression is violence. The point at the top of the anger triangle displays its integration center—will, motivation and determination. When expressed from its center, anger enables you to act from the highest truth: love.

Anger manifests in a wide range of unhealthy emotions. This includes, but is not limited to: fury, boredom, judgment, sarcasm, criticalness, cynicism, hostility, aggravation, rage, defiance, agitation, resistance, irritation, judgment, resentment, impatience, frustration, aggression, stubbornness, vengeance, hatred and bitterness.

Physical Characteristics of Anger

Physical characteristics that can indicate anger are erratic or labored breathing, shaking, a dry mouth, a red face, palpitation of the heart, muscular tension, headaches and difficulty calming down or relaxing.

Uncontrolled anger impairs the central nervous system's ability to function properly. It releases acid from the liver, which toxifies the blood and tissues and compromises the immune system, which makes you vulnerable to a wide variety of antigens. Uncontrolled anger also gives rise to a host of preventable dis-eases including hypertension, heart disease and TMJ, as well as a wide variety of cancers.

Anger Is Often Used to Mask Sadness

Masculine energy, in its natural capacity, acts to protect feminine energy. In relationship to emotions, anger—a masculine emotion—is expressed to hide, dismiss or deny the feminine emotion of sadness. Anger effectively keeps sadness from being exposed. For example, rather than admitting that being teased hurts and feels painful or embarrassing, you might react with anger.

This is one of the most destructive characteristics of anger.

As a reactive mechanism, anger can cause a great deal of emotional, mental or even physical harm. Anger keeps you oblivious to your own sadness, stopping you from identifying, acknowledging and feeling it. Turned inward, anger manifests as depression. Reactive anger can also manifest as passive/aggressive behavior, causing you to act out. In passive/aggressive behavior the sadness—in the form of pain, hurt or betrayal—is not openly admitted, but is displayed in covert angry reactions—retaliation, gossip, character assassination, punishment, lying and, in its most extreme display, violence.

Minimizing, Repressing, Dismissing or Denying Anger

While openly expressing anger causes great disturbances, the behaviors of denying, repressing, minimizing or dismissing anger is just as problematic, especially for women that are bound by societal protocols that deem the expression of anger as unacceptable. The consequences of this lack of acceptance manifest in these habitual, dis-ease-producing behaviors mentioned above that prevent you from finding a healthy outlet for the anger.

When anger is denied, minimized, repressed or dismissed, its energy accumulates in the emotional body and overflows into the mental body, where it causes obsessive, compulsive thoughts about the anger. When enough energy has accrued, it will implode—manifesting as depression—or explode—manifesting as violence.

Uncover the root cause of anger and you can transmute its

energy and eradicate angry reactions. This is the Radiant Key that will enable you to master anger's energy.

The Superficial Cause of Anger

Although the root cause of anger is fear, it does have a superficial cause, expectations.

Expectations are what you want, desire or expect to happen. Anger arises because an expectation has gone unfulfilled. For example, if you expect some money and do not get paid, or expect to have a favor returned and it is not, then anger will arise.

The greater the expectation, the greater the anger when the expectation is not met.

Identify expectations and you expose the root cause of anger. Release your expectations and you remove the possibility of anger. In turn you will flow through life's unexpected twists and turns with little pain and no suffering.

This is not an easy task, but it can be done.

Identify and release your expectations and the emotional energy of anger shifts away from the ego and into the center of the anger triangle. When you cannot find your expectations, the ego is rationalizing or justifying your behavior or actions. The ego wants to reinforce the belief that you are not responsible for your anger. It will try to convince you that someone else made you feel angry and therefore they are to blame. Deny responsibility for your anger and you will feel powerless and unable to change.

Remember: no one has the power to make you feel angry.

Vulnerability and Loss: The Core Fears behind Anger

While expectations are the sole cause of anger, the anger itself conceals two core fears: the fear of being vulnerable and the fear of loss. The two are discussed in detail in Chapter 25. For now, suffice to say that the ego also uses anger to conceal any emotion related to or arising from fear.

If you have learned that it is not okay to express your anger, then turn to Chapter 25 and read about Vulnerability and Loss. It can be extremely challenging to identify, own and express your anger in a healthy, direct and proactive way. However, it is possible.

You can harness anger's energy.

Reaching the Center of the Anger Triangle

When you experience frustration, aggravation or any other emotion attributed to anger's unhealthy range of expression, harness its energy and channel it into anger's healthy and productive center. Expressed from its center, anger's powerful energy is transformed into will, motivation and determination, and becomes the driving force that will enable you to accomplish any task or achieve any goal.

From its center, anger affects positive change.

Anger's energy can be used to uncover your expectations, change your attitude, perceptions, beliefs and behaviors, set boundaries, uncover your fears, express your feelings, ask for help, improve your communication or make amends. Take action from anger's center and you can overcome the unhealthy behaviors and habits that keep you from experiencing Radiant Health.

Seven Steps to Transmute Anger

The following seven steps will enable you to identify and own your anger, then transmute and express its energy in healthy ways. When you feel angry, put as many of these steps into action as you need.

Step 1. Identify Anger at Its Inception

Be honest with yourself when you feel angry. Identify the anger and accept its associated emotions, sensations and feelings. This major step towards emotional maturity gives you the opportunity to shift its energy from unhealthy to healthy.

Step 2. Practice Conscious Breathing Exercise #3

Do not act out your anger. Practice conscious breathing until its emotional energy subsides. In addition, take one or more of the following actions: pray to God to take your anger, and be willing to surrender it. Sing devotional songs to God, slowly drink a glass of room-temperature water to cool the fire of anger, lie down to keep the anger from rising, or slowly count backwards from ten to one as many times as needed until you feel calm.

Step 3. Identify Your Expectations and Desires

Be proactive. Do not react. Instead, turn your attention inward and uncover your expectations. Identify what you want or desire. People or events might push your "anger buttons," but you have the power to manage the energy. Expose the anger triggers and dismantle them.

Step 4. Do Not Speak until the Anger Subsides

Remain silent and practice conscious breathing. When the anger subsides and you have identified your expectations, use "I felt" statements to relate your desires, wants or fears. However, do not speak directly to the person involved; talk with a disinterested person. For example: *"I felt angry because I expected him to cook for me." "I felt angry because I expect to lose my job." "I felt angry because I do not want to feel vulnerable."* Ownership statements enable you to clearly express your feelings without blaming others for them.

Step 5. Take Responsibility for Your Anger

Own your anger, and its energy can empower you to change. Own your anger, and its energy becomes an unstoppable power that will drive you to achieve the goal of putting love into action.

Step 6. Transmute Anger's Energy to Will, Motivation and Determination

After identifying your expectations, bring the energy to anger's center and use it to create constructive, healthy goals. When Charles Atlas was young, he was bullied and beaten up because he was small. He harnessed his anger and used it to propel him towards his goal—to become a world champion body-builder. He transmuted his anger into motivation and determination and no one ever picked on him again.

Step 7. Be Open-Minded and Determined to Listen to Others

Anger often arises as a result of a miscommunication, misunderstanding or misperception. Listen to others' viewpoints. It takes honesty, integrity and courage to admit your part when you have become angry because of a misunderstanding. Admit your errors and your humility and self-respect improves.

Note: the essential oil from lavender can be used as a remedy to dissipate anger's energy. Lavender relaxes the muscles and tissues, and calms the mind. Put a few drops on a cloth, hold it a few inches from your nostrils and breathe in the aroma. Or, put a few drops of lavender oil into a small pot of boiled water, drape a towel over your head and slowly and carefully breathe in the steam.

Anger in Others

When anger arises in another, you might be able to help diffuse its destructive energy. First, drop your eyes so that you do not take in the anger energy. This is very important. Next, breathe deeply and be fully present. Remain silent and listen to what the angry person is saying. Do not agitate an angry person. Some people simply need to be heard and others need some time or space to cool off when they are angry. If you are asked to give some space, do it. Leave the room or house for a while. When you return, remain silent. If the person is calm and ready to talk listen quietly. If you are directly involved, do your best to not react. Take long deep breaths, listen carefully and try not to personalize the other person's feelings. Also, do not automatically assume responsibility if you are blamed. Honestly and introspectively look at your actions and, if your have erred, be mindful to admit your part.

Summation of Anger

Everyone experiences anger. Anger is part of the human emotional landscape. The key is to channel your anger into positive and healthy outlets. Be honest, introspective and willing to uncover your expectations. Put the seven steps into actions and the emotion of anger will provide you with rich opportunities for self-evaluation and personal growth. Take these steps and you will be putting love into action.

13

Sadness:
The Feminine Emotion

In the emotional body, sadness is the feminine counterpart to the masculine emotion, anger. Being able to embrace and experience them in equal measure is key to maintaining emotional balance and harmony. Because the repression or denial of sadness, tears or grief can lead to a wide variety of emotional, mental and physical dis-eases, this chapter contains exercises to help you express sadness. Before going further into the causes and effects of denied or repressed sadness, take a look at the sadness triangle.

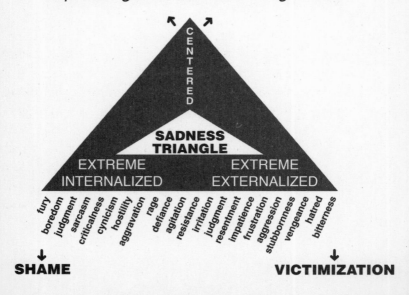

Honor Sadness
Expressing Grief and Shedding Tears

The Sadness Triangle Explained

At the base of the sadness triangle are its extreme polarities of unhealthy expression. Sadness's most Yin/internalized expression is shame, while its most Yang/externalized expression is victimization. The point at the top of the sadness triangle displays its integration center—embracing sadness by sharing grief and shedding tears.

Sadness also manifests in a wide range of unhealthy emotions. This includes, but is not limited to: martyrdom, guilt, rejection, hurt, sorrow, suffering, self-pity, embarrassment, disappointment, melancholy, self-deprecation, hopelessness, anguish, suffering, misery, remorse, loss and despair.

Sadness is related to the sensitive, tender, caring and vulnerable side of human nature. Openly expressing your sadness when it arises promotes healing, restores balance and preserves the integrity of the emotional, mental and physical bodies. When sadness is expressed from its center, the unhealthy polarities do not arise and the emotional body's creative energy flows unabated.

The key is to express your sadness candidly.

The Three Categories of Tears

Tears are one of the most candid expressions of sadness. There are three distinct categories of tears and they are ranked according to their emotional depth and level of intensity. Empathetic tears comprise the first category. Heart-tugging commercials and movie scenes, as well as dramatic and tragic human sagas, trigger them.

When empathetic tears are not related to a direct personal experience, they are low on the scale of intensity. If they parallel a direct personal experience, their intensity level increases and they are then ranked with either the second or third category of tears. In relationship to the senses, empathic tears have no distinguishing characteristics such as aroma, taste or sensation.

Tears of sadness constitute the second category. These tears are shed when you are experiencing personalized sadness. Feelings of guilt, disappointment, despair, rejection, shame and sorrow can provoke tears of sadness. Although tears of sadness have no distinct aroma or sensation, they do have one distinguishing sense-based quality—they have a salty flavor. Because tears of sadness promote greater healing, they rank higher on the scale than empathic tears.

Tears of grief comprise the final category. These tears arise in direct response to deep heart-felt pain and loss. Abandonment, death, abuse and long-standing suffering are some of the experiences that can evoke tears of grief. Because tears of grief are related to the most intense painful experiences, they are by far the most powerful, cleansing and health-producing tears.

A distinct odor, taste and sensation characterize tears of grief. The ammonia-like odor emitted by these tears represents long-held toxins being expelled from the body. Tears of grief have a bitter taste, and they sting the eyes. When all three physical characteristics—odor, taste and sensation—are present, they indicate deep heart-felt grief.

Tears Promote Holistic Health and Well-Being

Tears, when shed without hesitation or reservation, cleanse, purify and heal. They have a stimulating and harmonizing effect on the three bodies, and provide significant health-producing benefits. Physically, tears invigorate the immune system, eliminate toxins, reduce stress and tension and soothe the nerves. The need for rest and quiet is common after crying, and the cleansing properties of tears enable you to rest more comfortably and sleep more soundly.

Tears interrupt distractive mental body thoughts and analysis and narrow your focus and attention, bringing you fully into the present moment.

Tears effectively quiet the mind.

As tears silence the mind's mental chatter, the heart softens and sorrow, pain and grief melt away. Tears restore the free flow of creative energy to the emotional body. When tears are allowed to flow to completion, the dis-ease-producing energy from emotions such as frustration, anger, anxiety, agitation, fear and anguish dissolves. As the flow subsides, the natural harmonic resonance within the three bodies is reestablished. Laughter often follows, as feelings of peace and serenity return.

The release of tears leaves you feeling refreshed and alive.

The Sacred, Nurturing Power of Grieving

When the darkness of illusion is dispelled, experience dictates that Spirit exists in everything and death is an illusion. Nonetheless, that which has been loved and transitioned deserves to be grieved. This includes your relationships with family members, friends and pets and things like home and career. Experiences of abandonment, betrayal and abuse also need to be grieved, as does the loss of peace, security, innocence, safety, happiness and health.

Grieving is a testimony to love. It is a sacred, dignified and honorable way to express the distress of loss and relieve deep-seated pain and long-standing suffering. Grieving gives your heart a voice to praise that which has been lost. The high-pitched, heart-piercing sounds produced by wailing, screaming, howling and mourning vocalize the grief. Sobbing, moaning and weeping are softer forms used that expel grief.

The Healing Value of Grief Rituals

There is a proper way to grieve. As Mayan Shaman Martin Practael says, *"Grieving properly is where you look really bad when you are done; when your hair is missing and your clothes are ripped and you are down in the street."*[1]

To grieve properly is to fully let go.

Grief rituals are founded on feminine principles such as inclusion, nurturing and support. The purpose is to create a sacred container from which to express and purge the anguish, pain, hurt and despair of suffering and loss. Grief rituals bring individuals, families and communities into sacred contact with one another to harness the energy of pain and suffering and transform it into healing.

To grieve properly is to be supported.

Supported by family, friends and community, the griever opens the floodgates and dives into the heart-felt pain. Grieving is primal and chaotic. It does not follow rules of etiquette. The griever might cuss, scream and flail about in a state of hysteria.

To grieve properly is to be protected.

The griever's family, friends and community are sacred gatekeepers. When not directly affected, their job is to honor and maintain the sacredness and integrity of the grieving space. As the griever vocalizes the pain in his heart and curses his loss, it is the sacred gatekeepers' duty to keep him safe. They do not personalize his words or actions. They watch over him, keep him from hurting himself or others, give him food and water and provide for his every need. When his grieving concludes, which can last for days, weeks, months or longer, his family and friends welcome him back.

But in today's world, the sacred art of grieving has been lost.

How Grief Lost Its Sacred Place of Importance

With the advent of dominator cultures, the balance between masculine and feminine energy was annihilated. As the masculine model moved into a dominant role, it began the systematic destruction of the feminine model. Patriarchal religions, rituals and codes of behaviors were established. Feminine ritual, which honored everything as Spirit, and therefore part of the whole, was outlawed or destroyed. The patriarchy spun mythological tales that portrayed the feminine as being subservient to the masculine.

The face of the patriarchy is authoritarian, competitive, tough and staunchly independent. It has separated itself from the whole and therefore has no understanding or tolerance of feminine emotions. Over the last two thousand years the dominator mentality and its patriarchal dictates have become fortified in the collective consciousness. The foundation of modern social protocol and beliefs, with its roots firmly established in the darkness, lacks the experiential understanding that everything is Spirit. When the darkness is dissolved, balance will be reestablished.

Sadness will no longer be associated with weakness.

Honor and dignity will be restored to tears and grief.

Dominator Cultures Do Not Honor Grief

The feminine is generally treated with less dignity than the masculine. Thus, displays of tears and grief often have negative consequences like being teased and chastised, or judged as weak, cowardly, pitiful and disgusting, or being labeled a wimp, sissy or worse. The belief that crying is a display of weakness stops most people from being authentic when they are sad. This belief makes it extremely difficult, especially for boys and men, to openly cry, to support and nurture or provide compassion and understanding to those who are grieving. The belief that you are weak if you cry will cause you to feel guilty and ashamed of grief, and cause you to deny pain.

But sadness, tears and grief are part of the human experience.

Human beings are emotional by nature. Tragically, feminine emotions are not honored and supported. Those who display pain are judged and condemned, while those who internalize it are honored and praised. Messages like "pull yourself up by the bootstraps," "suck it up" and "don't let nothing get you down" characterize the dominator mentality. They are indicative of a dogged determination to avoid feeling or showing pain. But the air of invincibility conveyed by these messages contradicts the destructive nature of repressed sadness, tears and grief. The messages also discount the true strength it takes to openly express grief.

The Overflowing Burden Basket of Grief

People today are burdened by an overwhelming amount of grief. And it is not just their own. They have inherited the grief of their parents, grandparents and great-grandparents. They carry the grief of entire generations of people who were subject to massacres, slavery and genocide. Those who died as a result of the violence perpetuated by the dominator culture have not been properly grieved.

When grief is not expressed, its energy builds.

When the pain and suffering in the hearts and minds of the conquered is not grieved, it is transferred to their offspring. With each passing generation, the burden of unexpressed grief grows larger and heavier. In cases of genocide, the vibrations of pain and suffering hover in the ethers and are held in the land where they died. Until the grief is expressed the toxic vibrations will continue to saturate the heart, mind and body, producing deadly dis-eases. Grieving honors the pain and suffering of the ancestors, cleanses the land, feeds the spirits and expels the toxins that cause physical, mental and emotional dis-ease.

Withheld Sadness, Tears and Grief Leads to Dis-ease

Heart dis-ease and lower back pain are two of the highest ranked dis-eases in the nation. These front runners of modern dis-ease have a causal relationship to unexpressed sadness, tears and grief. The epidemic of heart dis-ease and lower back pain is a sign that the burden basket of grief has been filled beyond capacity. If the burden basket continues to overflow it will be passed down to our children, and they will suffer.

The heart is the metaphysical organ related to love. While modern medical practitioners might point to poor diet, stress or a sedentary lifestyle as the common indicators of heart dis-ease, feeling unloved is the primary factor that is at the root of this dis-ease. Lower back pain relates to feeling a lack of emotional support. Because dominator cultures do not honor feminine rituals and emotions, the lower back becomes the repository for sadness, tears and grief.

Heart dis-ease and lower back pain affect men in far greater numbers than women. This is no surprise considering men are not supported to openly express their sadness. According to the dictates of a patriarchal society his sadness must be carried stoically. The adage "a man's gotta do what a man's gotta do" is a prime example of the dominator mentality. Because of this mentality, most men and even some women are not comfortable with expressions of sadness or love, which include support and nurturing. When the need to be supported or nurtured arises, it creates intense discomfort.

The energy it takes to withhold sadness weakens the immune system, can cause a loss of appetite and leaves you feeling sluggish, drained and exhausted. Eventually, the joints begin to ache, muscles atrophy and organs malfunction. The energy of unexpressed sadness also affects the psyche. It can manifest in emotional and mental dis-eases including alcoholism, drug addiction, depression, obsessions, compulsions and breakdowns. Unexpressed grief gives rise to intense internalized feelings such as loneliness, emptiness, isolation and depression.

Today, unexpressed grief is erupting in the form of deadly violence. As stated in Hopi prophecy, Chapter 2, "Children will be out of control and will no longer obey the leaders." This prophecy is being fulfilled with startling accuracy as the masculine emotion, anger, is used to mask the feminine emotion, sadness.

Violence is a representation of unexpressed grief.

As a direct result of being afraid to express sadness, anger is used to protect its feminine counterpart. Anger rises in direction proportion to the level of fear one has in experiencing sadness. When unexpressed grief reaches the saturation point, anger rises up and is expressed in one of its extremes—suicide or violence, or deadly dis-ease. Long-term unexpressed grief can manifest in any number of cancers, which indicates unexpressed anger, which in turn is a disguise for sadness and grief. The lethal results of repressed sadness have been witnessed at Columbine High and other schools and neighborhoods around the country.

Boys are most vulnerable.

Boys Are Victimized by Unexpressed Sadness

The alarming frequency of destructive fits of violence from boys results in part from routine overt and covert messages that it is not okay to express sadness. Boys who get the message that it is not manly or acceptable to cry learn to withhold their tears and internalize their sadness. The withheld sadness festers, and, without a safe way to express it, eventually erupts in rage. The rage has now pushed beyond social norms of arguing and fighting, and has escalated into deadly acts of violence.

Boys who learn to withhold their tears grow into adults who have trouble being vulnerable. These boys build protective walls around their hearts, and do not share their feelings. They do not trust. As the heart's armor gets thicker the tears are transformed into acts of violence or manifest as tumors.

Boys are in desperate need of grief rituals.

The issue of expressing sadness and grief in a healthy manner will be addressed and resolved when men courageously open their hearts, step forward and take the following three actions.

1. **Examine**. Examine what you have been taught, what you believe and what you teach others, through your actions, about expressing sadness.

2. **Change**. Make a commitment to yourself, your family—especially to your son or boys in your community—and other men to openly express your sadness and support them when they are sad.

3. **Heal**. Pray for guidance. Ask Spirit to help you create a sacred space to perform a grief ceremony. Initially, invite men, and later boys, to participate; return to the traumas and losses which have not been grieved. Honor and support others as they grieve. Allow others to support you as you grieve.

Common Obstacles That Impede Expressing Sadness

Being judged as weak, being consumed or immobilized by grief, crying buckets of tears or drowning in sorrow are common fears that lead to the internalization of sadness. Trying to figure out why you feel sad is another major obstacle. As the energy is transferred from the emotional body to the mental body, feeling the sadness recedes and thinking about the sadness takes over.

The more you analyze, the less you feel.

Do not think first—feel first.

After the tears subside, the cause of the sadness will often rise to the surface. If it does not, do not try to figure it out. Often there are no rational explanations. Lunar cycles, somatic memory and other anomalies can trigger bouts of sadness. As a sentient, Spirit being, you are sensitive to all energies. The vibrations of ungrieved pain in your family members, friends and the collective consciousness can trigger sadness.

Reaching the Center of the Sadness Triangle

When you experience sadness or any other emotion on the sadness scale, put the following steps into action.

Step 1. When You Feel Sad, Stop What You Are Doing.

Be quiet. Turn your focus and attention inward. Focus the mind on conscious breathing exercise #1. Breathe into the sadness.

Step 2. Do Not Invalidate Your Own or Anyone Else's Sadness.

Sadness and tears are often judged and ridiculed, so be mindful not to invalidate your sadness. Do not laugh, shut it off or talk your way through it. Remind yourself that there is nothing wrong with crying. If you feel uncomfortable be still. Being still might seem to be passive, but it is an active way to allow the sadness to rise. You are not "doing nothing," but rather creating a sacred, safe, nurturing and supportive container for yourself and others to express sadness.

Step 3. Be Patient. Do Not Distract Yourself.

Relax into your sadness and feel it. Affirm that it is okay to be sad. Do not analyze or resist it. When any distracting thought form pops up—sadness often stimulates distracting thoughts—focus on conscious breathing. Otherwise, you risk talking through the sadness rather than feeling it. If tears do not come immediately, do not

eat, watch TV, play loud music, talk, get angry or do anything else
to avoid the sadness.

Be patient, mindful and quiet until the tears arise.

Step 4. Share Your Sadness, Tears and Grief with Others.

"Joy shared is multiplied and pain shared is divided" is a popular
adage. When you feel sad, share it with a close trustworthy friend.
Sharing sadness is one way to create a supportive and nurturing
environment. The thought might arise, "There is no one I can trust."
This is the ego's way to try to hide the sadness. Do not give thoughts
of these kinds attention. Instead, pray for help and ask for support.
Ask friends that you trust to honor your sadness by providing a quiet
space, lending a shoulder to lean on, not talking until you are ready
and being ready to listen. The quieter the mind and environment is,
the fewer the distractions and the greater the opportunity to express
and release the sadness.

Step 5. Ask to Be Nurtured.

It can be very challenging to receive love and support when you
feel sad. This is especially true if you have been taught that it is not
okay to ask for help. Allow others to create a safe and nurturing
space for you. Open your heart and feel the warmth and care that
come from being hugged or held while you are crying. When the
tears have been fully released, you will have a new perspective on
your experiences. You will feel replenished, refreshed, lighter and
energized. Spontaneous laughter often follows the release of sadness. Afterwards, take some quiet time, have a light snack or a cup
of tea.

Step 6. Create a Nurturing Environment for Others.

When someone else feels sad, create a safe space for him/her to
experience it. Be mindful of your own feelings. If you feel uncomfortable, practice conscious breathing exercise #1 and be still. Do
not deny, minimize or invalidate another person's sadness. Open
your heart and support him/her. Bring honor and dignity to the
process by being a sacred gatekeeper for the sadness.

14

Laughter: The Emotion of the Divine Child

Although laughter is the defining emotion of the Divine Child, expressing anger or sadness from its center is in alignment with the Divine Child's nature. Healthy emotional expression indicates conscious awareness and represents the authentic nature of the Divine Child. However, when it comes to emotions, laughter emits a vibration resonant to that of love.

As an emotion, laughter has incredible healing properties. Laughter and tears are the only two non-food substances that stimulate, activate and energize your immune system. In *Anatomy of an Illness*, Norman Cousins wrote of the prominent role that laughter played in healing him of a life-threatening dis-ease.

Laughter Heals a Dying Man

After a jam-packed trip abroad, Norman returned home with a slight fever that soon escalated to a full-blown illness. His sickness was marked by difficulty in moving his neck, arms, hands, fingers and legs. Within a week of being home, Norman was hospitalized.

Norman's sedimentation rate[1] had reached 88, and within another week it was up to 115—a reading associated with a critical condition. Several specialists were called and they all concurred that Norman was suffering from a serious collagen dis-ease. The prognosis was dim. He was given a one in five hundred chance of full recovery. One specialist stated that he had never personally witnessed anyone recover from the severity of Norman's condition.

His condition was believed to be terminal.

Neither the doctors' prognosis nor their lack of confidence in his ability to recover would sway Norman. He had always firmly believed that laughter had a salutary effect on one's health and well-being. Armed with numerous written works of humor, producer Alan Funt's *Candid Camera* series and Marx Brothers films, Norman began the journey to laugh himself to recovery. He also enlisted vitamin C for his fight, and the help of his close friend Dr. William Hitzig.

Norman always believed in the body's own natural power and ability to heal itself. With a positive, proactive attitude, and an unshakable belief in his ability to get well, Norman devoted himself full-time to laughter. He undertook the challenge to become the first person in recorded history to prove the healing effects of laughter.

At Norman's request, Dr. Hitzig would run sedimentation rate tests on him just before and several hours after the laughing episodes. Each time Norman was tested after a prolonged episode of laughter, Dr. Hitzig noted a drop of five points in the sedimentation rate. The change, although not dramatic, was cumulative. By the end of the eighth day, Norman's sedimentation rate was somewhere in the 80s and dropping fast.

It took him many months to regain his mobility and even longer to become almost completely pain-free. But Norman's scientifically documented story of laughing his way back to health provides a bright ray of hope for those diagnosed with chronic or seemingly terminal dis-eases.

Destructive Forms of Laughter

Some forms of humor display a lack of humility and maturity. Sarcasm is a biting, scathing humor that encourages laughter at another person's expense. Some people tease and ridicule others to gain attention. Ridiculing others might make you laugh, but the person who is the brunt of the joke does not share in the laughter.

Teasing children can inflict deep, lasting emotional wounds and damage their self-esteem. Sometimes people laugh to disguise emotions. For example, if you laugh at someone who is in pain, this can indicate your unexpressed anger, discomfort with expressing sadness or inability to empathize with pain.

The Scientific Healing Effects of Laughter

The Western medical establishment has documented the scientific healing effects of laughter. For example, hearty laughter increases the secretions of endorphins, which in turn increases the oxygenation of the blood, speeds up the heart, relaxes the arteries and decreases blood pressure. Laughter also has a positive effect on all cardiovascular and respiratory ailments, as well as increasing the overall immune system response.

Laughter is a powerful reducer of stress and tension.

Episodes of laughter often follow the release of intense emotions. Laughter is a great mood stabilizer and mood changer. It requires no prescription, has no negative side effects and is a great way to open your heart. Laughing does not cost anything and can restore you to holistic health.

The more laughter you bring to your home, work, community, relationships and life the healthier you will be. The more you laugh, the happier and more satisfied you will feel. Be willing to laugh at yourself, and do not take yourself or life so seriously. Be silly. Wear a crown and cape or a rainbow Afro wig to work. Laugh until you cry, and your immune system's response ability doubles.

Open your heart and mind to the humor in everyday life. You will feel lighter, and your hearty laughter will make you a likely candidate to achieve Radiant Health and maintain it.

15

Passion

The word *passion* arises from the Latin word *passius*, which means "to suffer." Passion is relegated to the outer layer of the emotional body because its energy, like all outer layer components, can be controlled by the ego or governed by the heart. Fire, which is the gross energy of passion, must always be handled with great care and awareness, because while fire can purify, it can also destroy. And indeed, the fiery energy of passion often falls prey to the ego, which can cause terrible damage and tremendous suffering.

Ego-Driven Passion

The ego ignites the destructive flames of passion. Fueled by the ego, passion's fiery energy turns chaotic, scorching everything in its path. Ego-driven passions are characterized by a seeming lack of concern for one's own health and well-being, as well as the health and well-being of others. Ego-driven passions are marked by selfishness, ignorance, greed, over-indulgence and a lack of vision for the greater good.

Ego-driven passions have one common denominator: they mask an unfulfilled Spirit.

You, as Spirit, took a human form to fulfill a specific Spiritual purpose. If, however, you do not realize that you are Spirit, then the constructive flames of passion, which support your inward drive and focus to find and carry out your Spiritual purpose, become destructive. Without a clearly established Spiritual focus and purpose for your life, the ego seizes the fiery energy of passion and directs it outward to the world of sensual and material fulfillment.

Captured by the ego, passion's fire becomes addictions and obsessions.

Addictions and obsessions are marked by a constant craving for sensual pleasure, stimulation, excitement, adventure or control. To satisfy the insatiable, all-consuming fire of an addiction or obsession becomes a full-time job. But feeding it provides only temporary satisfaction. As the desire for greater stimulation and gratification escalates, the addiction or obsession demands more of your time and energy.

Ego-driven passions lead to a dead-end road.

Addictions and obsessions destroy clear thinking. Healthy qualities such as motivation, acceptance, sacrifice, compassion, forgiveness, dignity, patience, integrity and honesty fall by the wayside. The ability to manage emotions is also seriously impaired. Addictions and obsessions disguise the deep heartache, pain and suffering produced by a lack of Spiritual awareness and focus. In the end, addictions and obsessions rob you of your emotional, mental and physical health and well-being, leave you feeling empty, alone and depressed.

But the fire of passion can also be used constructively.

Heart-Driven Passion

When passion's fire arises from the heart, its focus is directed towards God and the realization that *You are God*. Heart-driven passion is a positive force that provides you with boundless energy, propelling you to greater conscious awareness and ultimately Radiant Health. Steered by the heart, passion's fire drives you to realize your own divinity, and recognize and acknowledge the divinity inherent in each and every living thing. Passion's fire sparks creativity, imagination, innovation, inspiration, enthusiasm, excitement and adventure. When directed by the heart, passion's fire brings you into direct alignment with the Divine, providing all the energy you need to put *Love into Action* and experience Radiant Health.

Driven by your heart, the fire of passion energizes and inspires you to annihilate the ego and its illusions of separation, so that you can recognize and embrace your true nature. The fire of heart-driven passion warms your soul, makes you feel alive, expands your conscious awareness and drives you to experience yourself and others as God. Heart-driven passion provides the fire to heal wounds, put *Love and Truth in Action*, bring your life's purpose to light, inspire your prayers and fuel your *Journey to Radiant Health*.

Heart-driven passion propels you to self-realization.

When used in conjunction with its mental body counterpart, Will—see Chapter 23—heart-driven passion rises to an even higher level. Both passion and Will are fire energies; passion being feminine and Will being masculine. When brought together, your creative fire becomes crystal clear and laser sharp. The feminine and masculine fires purify your vision, burn away ego impurities like fear, worry, negativity, procrastination and impatience and energize your efforts to experience Radiant Health.

The fire of heart-driven passion gives you the energy, initiative and enthusiasm to discard destructive habits and institute healthy change. Heart-driven passion fuels your Spiritual growth. It infuses you with healthy, creative and exciting ideas, and fills your heart with joy, gratitude and satisfaction.

Heart-driven passion is always in alignment with your life's purpose. Its energy enables you to embrace Spirit; nurture, support and serve those in need; and achieve the higher goal of self-realization.

HEART-DRIVEN PASSION EXERCISE I
Write down everything that makes you feel passionate.

Think of everything that makes you feel passionate. This might include being with animals, reading, teaching children, walking on the beach, playing baseball, talking about Spirituality or practicing meditation. Do not limit yourself. Keep the list handy; you will need to use it in the next exercise.

HEART-DRIVEN PASSION EXERCISE II

Use your heart-driven passion to put Love into Action.

Whenever you feel dull, listless, uninspired or apathetic, take out your list of things that make you feel passionate. Use the fire of heart-driven passion to put something on the list into action. Make a conscious choice to see God in all of creation and put Love into Action. Open your eyes really wide, bring a great big smile to your face and acknowledge your own Divinity. Allow the fire of heart-driven passion to alter the way you feel.

-16-

Experiences

Experiences, especially those that occur during childhood, shape your belief systems, attitudes and perceptions. Whether healthy or unhealthy, they play a major role in determining how you view life and the world, and how you identify yourself.

Although you can not change your experiences, you can change your attitude towards them. It is possible to find light in even the darkest experience, and use even the most pain-filled experiences as a springboard to Spiritual growth and healing. When healing takes place, experiences can be put into the proper perspective, and then you can use them as a tool to inspire others to embark on a path of healing.

Imprinting

Every experience in life is stored in the subtle energy astral body—which contains the emotional and mental bodies—and in the gross physical body. Although the mental body stores experiences as memories and the emotional body stores experiences as feelings, the physical body is the primary container for all experiences. Each cell in the physical body stores information. Like a sponge, each cell absorbs the subtle thought-form and emotion energies from the mental and emotional bodies, as well as the physical sensations from an experience.

As the energy is absorbed, it causes an imprint.

Imprinting occurs when an experience produces an intense sensation—typically described as pleasure or pain. When an experience produces an intense sensation, an electro-magnetic charge is imprinted, which results in craving or aversion. The subtle emotional and mental electro-magnetic charge is imprinted in the gross physical body, which stores the information in its cells.

The word *attachment* is synonymous with imprint.

When a current event mirrors a previous experience, the imprint (the original sensation associated with the past experience) is triggered, causing you to react. Produced by fear, reactions give rise to unhealthy emotions such as rage, lust, anxiety, impatience, envy, resentment, worry, hysteria and guilt, as well as unhealthy behaviors such as blame, criticism, co-dependency, judgment, expectations, sentimentality, worship, addictions, compulsions or obsessions, arrogance or deceit.

The stronger the imprint/attachment, the stronger the reaction.

Fear produces reactions, such as resistance and desire. When an imprint is triggered, the resistance to feel pain or the desire to feel pleasure causes you to react. Reaction leads to resistance—when the fear is that you will feel pain. Reaction leads to desire—when the fear is that you will *not* feel (enough) pleasure.

Healing occurs when energetic imprints are discharged.

Discharge imprints/attachments and you will live in Bliss, fully present in every moment.

Physical Imprints

The ramifications of imprinting are unique to each body. Emotional, mental or physical trauma or abuse causes intense sensation. The most common reaction to intense sensation is to hold the breath and tense the body. Reaction imprints the sensation in the cells, specifically imprinting the reactive energy into the cells in the part of the body being clenched such as the jaw, back, shoulders, neck, buttocks, hands, etc. If emotions (anger or sadness) are stifled during the experience, their energy also will be imprinted in the physical cells of the part of the body being tensed. The pleasure associated with activities that stimulate the five senses—touch, taste, sound, sight and smell—such as eating, exercise, sex, music, alcohol or drugs for example, can also imprint an electro-magnetic charge in the physical body's cells.

Physical imprints can be dissolved.

Dissolving Physical Imprints

When you experience acute or chronic pain in a specific part of the body for no ostensible reason, it might be related to an imprint. Deep-tissue massage, Rolfing, Rebirthing (the breath-work developed by Leonard Orr), Acupressure, Reiki, Chi-Gong and Cranial Sacral Therapy are bodywork techniques that are extremely effective in identifying and releasing subtle energetic emotional or mental imprints lodged in the physical body. The ability to release imprints makes bodywork essential on *The Journey to Radiant Health*. Keep in mind that the majority of physical dis-eases have an emotional cause. The Index contains a list of physical dis-eases and the emotional root for each.

Mental Imprints

In the mental body, imprints can cause you to link current events to past memories. For example, if you suffered abuse at the hands of an authority figure in the past, then dealing with an authority figure in the present is likely to trigger the imprint. The memories rise to the surface, cause you to worry or feel anxious and fearful, and affect your ability to be calm and confident during the interaction.

Imprints adversely affect your ability to maintain mental clarity, focus and concentration, and can cause you to feel a range of emotions from discomfort to insecurity to paralyzing fear. Imprints can also cause you to feel self-conscious, overanalyze events, second-guess yourself or put unnecessary pressure on yourself when you need to make an important decision. Imprints can cause you to obsess on past pleasures or pains, which robs you of being fully present in the moment. Imprints can also keep you from facing uncomfortable feelings.

Mental imprints produce a variety of dis-eases including confusion, obsessions, attachments, cravings, aversions, worry, daydreams and nightmares, regrets, longing, restlessness, compulsions and addictions. Mental body dis-eases are rooted in reliving past events or projecting fear into future possibilities.

Mental imprints can be dissolved.

Dissolving Mental Imprints

To dissolve electro-magnetic charges imprinted in the mental body, put the following technique into action.

1. Bring the imprinted memory causing the mental dis-ease to mind. The memory brought to mind will have an emotional charge.

2. Run the event through your mind from beginning to end. Take a heated argument with a colleague for example. Start at the beginning of the argument and run it one time through your mind from beginning to end.

3. Re-frame the memory. This time, start at the beginning of the argument and re-frame the entire memory. For example, as the argument begins, change his facial features: see his ear growing bigger, his nose getting longer and his eyes bulging out like a cartoon character. As the scene continues, shrink him to the size of a small child and pat him on the head, or put him into a clown suit with a red nose and big floppy shoes.

4. Run the re-framed event from beginning to end.

5. Reverse the process and run the re-framed event from end to beginning.

Repeat steps 4 and 5. Run the event forward and backward until the memory can be consistently brought to mind with the new framing intact. When the technique has been implemented effectively the imprinted emotional charge will be dissolved, and the new framing will produce laughter.

Note: Do not use this technique in a current or ongoing emotional situation, or in lieu of expressing your emotions.

Emotional Imprints

Although electro-magnetic charges can be imprinted during any experience, the charges imprinted during childhood often have the greatest impact on your life because they strongly influence the belief systems, attitudes and perceptions you adopt about yourself, other people, places and life in general.

Imprints of Childhood Abuse

Children who experience emotional, mental or physical abuse suffer low self-esteem, engage in self-sabotaging reactive emotions and behaviors and lack the ability to trust. The abuse transforms a child's creative emotional energy from healthy to unhealthy, stunting his emotional growth and maturing process.

Abused children often act out or are destructive and defiant. They do not act out because they are inherently "bad" but because the only attention they have ever received is "negative attention." It is very challenging to overcome the depth and severity of imprints that result from childhood abuse. The odds are heavily stacked against an abused child growing up to be an emotionally healthy adult.

But it can be done.

Identifying Abusive Experiences

The first step is to identify abuse; being hit with objects, spanked or slapped are obvious forms of physical abuse, but emotional and mental abuse is just as harmful and often more subtle. Consider the example of an injured child. A child falls and skins her knee. She seeks the safety and comfort of Mom's love. But, instead of being nurtured, she is scolded or told, "It's not that bad," "Big girls don't cry," "Can't you do anything right?" or "You are such a klutz."

In the example, the child experienced an injury, pain and fear. She needed comfort, love and compassion, but her mother reacted with anger, irritation and disappointment. The difference between what the child experienced and her mother's reaction can cause the child to feel confused. If her mother's reactive behavior continues, the child will begin to question whether her own authentic emotions are valid. In time, the child will shut down emotionally and begin acting out the dysfunctional behavior patterns of her mother.

The mother might be treating her daughter the same way she was treated as a child. The mother's unhealed childhood wounds cause her to perpetuate the pattern of abuse. She is unaware of the negative impact her behavior has on her child's emotional health and well-being. The mother does not comfort her child, nor does she give her child any positive, supportive messages.

This is an example of emotional and mental abuse.

Not meeting a child's emotional needs—such as being heard, nurtured, supported or acknowledged—constitutes subtle emotional and mental abuse. Minimizing, dismissing or treating her physical wounds with scorn and indignation constitutes blatant emotional and mental abuse.

Child Abuse Causes Dysfunctional Adult Behaviors

It is not unusual for children who experience subtle or blatant abuse to decide that it is unsafe to share their pain with others. Fearing reprisal, they learn to hide their feelings. Until their emotional wounds are treated and healed, the fear of being attacked will make it difficult for them to be authentic, share from the heart or take risks.

Abused children generally grow into emotionally stifled adults.

Being honest and emotionally open is difficult. Co-dependent behaviors such as repressing or denying emotions become common, especially if it is believed that being emotionally authentic will upset someone. Emotionally and mentally abused adult children suffer from low self-esteem, often believing that they are inadequate or unworthy of love.

Destructive behaviors reflect a lack of self-love and respect. They include fighting, self-mutilation and eating disorders like bulimia and anorexia, as well as self-deprecation, expressing emotions without boundaries or acting out inappropriately to get attention.

These behaviors are a sign of stifled emotional growth.

Many adults are unaware that what they experienced as a child qualifies as abuse. Adults often minimize the abuse they experienced with dismissive statements like "It was no big deal," "I was a bad kid," "I deserved to be hit" or "Other kids had it a lot worse than me." These statements also illustrate the difficulty in being characterized as a victim of abuse.

No one wants to be labeled a victim.

Yet, when a child experiences abuse, they learn that love is synonymous with pain and suffering. The legacy of an adult who has not healed his own emotional and mental wounds is that of the abused child that grows up to be an abuser.

Unravel and Dissolve Unhealthy Imprints

The negative charges associated with dysfunctional imprints and conditioning do not have to rule your life. You do not have to become the culmination of your experiences. You do not have to be a victim. You are Spirit and you can change. You have the power, and ultimately the freedom, to make conscious choices that will facilitate healing. You can unravel unhealthy imprints and reconnect to the light of your Divine nature.

When you heal the wounds of childhood abuse, the negative imprints will dissolve. Your self-esteem will improve and you will begin to trust and follow your inner guidance. Dysfunctional behavior patterns will dissolve, you will become less reactive, and you will come to understand that you do matter, you are important and you are a Divine child of Spirit.

You will realize you are lovable and worthy of being loved.

Your social and intimate relationships will improve. You will begin to treat yourself and others with more kindness, care, compassion and consideration. Your listening skills will improve and you will sense when others are in pain. Then, rather than reacting to their actions and behaviors, you will act to help them.

Heal your wounds and you will break the cycle of re-creating the past abuse. By doing this you will break the chains of familial, cultural, racial, national and ancestral dysfunction.

When the experiences at hand cause painful past events to resurface they also present you with an opportunity to change your attitudes, beliefs and perceptions. The process of unraveling imprints begins by putting the first five steps on *The Journey to Radiant Health* into practice. Start with step one, *Conscious Breathing,* to turn your attention inward and increase your conscious awareness. Next, practice step two, *Put Love into Action,* to uncover that which is resistant to Love—all emotional and mental imprints create feelings, thoughts that are resistant to Love. Step three, *Pray and Meditate Every Day,* will magnetize the Divine to you, providing the guidance, strength and support you will need to change. Step four, *Develop a Relationship with Your Spirit Child*—which you will discover in Chapter 17— will help you identify and heal long-standing wounds. The practice of step five, *Be Honest and Truthful in All your Affairs,* will transform unhealthy behaviors and belief systems to healthy ones.

Practice the first five steps on *The Journey to Radiant Health,* and the emotional, mental and physical imprinted charges will dissipate, and you will be less inclined to react when memories, feelings or events arise that remind you of the past. The final step is to maintain vigilance—which is best accomplished by continuing to work with conscious breathing—over any thoughts and emotions that arise in relationship to present events, so that you recognize and dissolve any remaining imprints that catapult you into the past or propel you into the future, and stop you from being completely present in the here and now.

Healthy, Loving Experiences

In the previous example, an injured child was not treated with love or compassion. Now imagine the same scene with a healthy outcome. The child falls and injures herself. She feels pain and fear, and begins to cry. Then she finds a parent/authority figure that listens to her story, comforts her and tends to her wound. Having been heard and acknowledged, she soon feels better and resumes her activities. She knows her emotions are valid and she feels confident sharing them.

Healing childhood wounds will enable you to model healthy behaviors. In Chapter 17, you will have the opportunity to meet your Spirit Child and start the process to identify and heal your childhood wounds. The Spirit Child will help you bring light to the darkness of abuse and trauma.

Then you can take action to dissolve your imprints.

Using Step Three, "Pray and Meditate Every Day," to Support Detachment

Prayer and meditation are cornerstones that strengthen your ability to detach from reactions. A simply phrased prayer, such as "help me detach from this anger," repeated consistently with heart-driven passion, can dissipate reactive energy.

After the mind is saturated with the prayer, follow it with meditation. Begin your meditation by focusing on the breath. This will help to quiet the mind. Next, bring your attention to the heart and open it to the energy of Love. Be receptive to the guidance that comes from Spirit, your Angels and Guides. As you learn to follow your inner guidance, you will discover that it provides you with answers that enable you to put love and truth in action.

-17-

The Spirit Child:
Portal to Shamanism,
Soul Retrieval and Healing

The soul contains our vital essence and is the central hub that acts as the integrating point for the three bodies. Soul loss is an ancient term that describes the Spiritual origin of illness and dis-ease. Soul loss typically occurs as a result of traumas such as the loss of a loved one, a severe injury or accident, surgery, sexual abuse, chronic or acute stress or illness, violent assault or other abuse, and gives rise to varying degrees of emotional, mental and physical disorders.

In a Spiritual context, what occurs is that part of the soul "splits off" to ensure that the individual survives the intense and often unbearable pain associated with the traumatic episode. While experiencing the trauma the victim often simultaneously recalls witnessing the event from a distant vantage point beyond the body, bearing evidence of the soul's departure.

When a part of the soul splits off, a void is left.

Soul loss is an epidemic in Western civilization, yet medicine, psychology and psychiatry do not recognize it as a precursor for disease. Nonetheless the medical and mental sciences have unknowingly categorized and described soul loss's most common effects. Emotional and mental disorders such as anxiety, bulimia, anorexia, phobia, depression, addiction, mania, schizophrenia, obsessive/compulsive, hyperactivity, bi-polar, attention deficit and many others are a by-product of soul loss. The void left by the departure of part of the soul requires something to fill it, which is, most often, some form of dis-ease. Victims of soul loss can also be described as "having a vacant look in the eyes," "being an empty shell" or "being possessed." Possession takes place when the void, created by the soul's departure from the astral body, is filled by a disincarnate being—a soul that does not have a body.

Scientific evidence, which is essential to accept soul loss as being a valid precursor to dis-ease, is not available because the soul's existence cannot be proven. Because Western medical models are bound by the limitations of science, they cannot accept soul loss as a valid explanation for emotional, mental and physical dis-ease. Hence, they are limited to defining and treating the superficial symptoms of soul loss—emotional and mental disorders—without being able to uncover and heal their true root cause.

Treating symptoms does not facilitate core-level healing.

There is, however, an ancient practice that does.

Shamanism

For tens of thousands of years the Spiritual origins of dis-ease have been treated using a potent and effective model, Shamanism. The word *Shaman* traces back to the Tungas tribe in Siberia and means "one who sees in the dark." In tribal culture, when an individual suffers from an emotional, mental or physical illness, in addition to treating the visible symptoms, a Shaman is summoned to journey to the Spirit world to ascertain the Spiritual cause.

Traditionally, the Shaman uses rhythmic drumming, or in very rare cases psychotropic substances, to enter an altered state of conscious awareness, which provides access to the non-ordinary reality of the Spirit realm. After permission is granted by the afflicted individual, the Shaman can journey to the Spirit realm to ascertain the Spiritual nature and origins of the disorder. The Shaman directly intervenes in the healing process by using teachers, guides and power animals from the Spirit world to search for the missing fragment of the soul, locate it and return it to the individual.

This ancient healing technique is called *"Soul Retrieval."*

Treat Dis-ease or Heal Dis-ease?

Contemporary models for treating dis-ease have long dismissed, as superstition, the beliefs of indigenous peoples in the power of Shamans to facilitate healing. A dramatic rise in conscious awareness as well as the failure of science, psychotherapy and medicine to develop effective methods for healing, however, has led more and more people to return to the ancient tradition of Shamanism. This Spiritual renaissance has led to a resurgence in the interest and exploration of the mysterious, ancient and yet highly effective, time-tested healing practice of Shamanism. The Spirit Child can guide you to the non-ordinary reality of the Spirit realm and, when its guidance is followed meticulously, can help you perform your own Soul Retrieval.

The Spirit Child

The second layer of the emotional body is home to the Spirit Child. Developing a relationship with the Spirit Child is a stepping stone to reestablishing the connection to your own Spirit—the Divine Child, which is created by the merging of your feminine and masculine energy. Although the Spirit Child is not a classic shamanic tool used to perform Soul Retrieval, it does reside in the non-ordinary realm of Spirit and is capable of assisting you to reclaim soul fragments. To make contact with the Spirit Child it is essential to have an open mind. Be willing to venture beyond the belief systems and structures that limit the mind's perceptions to ordinary reality. Developing a relationship with the Spirit Child—the fourth step on *The Journey to Radiant Health*—is essential to the recovery, healing and integration of all aspects of the self.

You, the Spirit Realm and Balance

A child naturally possesses the ability to move fluidly between the ordinary material world and the non-ordinary Spirit world. As a child grows older, however, she is socialized, indoctrinated into limited, dogmatic systems that teach her to classify that which exists outside the boundaries of the material world as imagination, or even as dangerous and evil. When the natural connection between a child and the Spirit world is severed, imbalance occurs.

One way to reestablish your organic connection with the Spirit world is to meet your Spirit Child. Renewing this bond can resolve the Cartesian split and return the heart and mind, and feminine and masculine, to a natural harmonic state of balance. The Spirit Child can gently reintroduce you to the realm of Spirit, providing you with information that can promote emotional, mental or physical healing. Continual interaction with the Spirit Child will enable you to recognize and acknowledge it as a valid, integral and important part of your awareness, growth and healing.

In this chapter you will find a simple, time-tested meditation technique that will enable you to relax your body and enter a state of altered consciousness from which you can meet your own Spirit Child and have your own personal experience with the Spirit realm. If you are not comfortable or ready to experience the Spirit realm, you are unlikely to meet the Spirit Child. This is okay. Do not judge yourself. To explore the Spirit world with an open mind requires letting go of fearful imprints, belief systems and dogmas surrounding non-ordinary reality. If you are ready, then the Spirit Child can become your ally. As the gatekeeper to the heart, it will help you begin the process of learning to listen to your inner guidance. The Spirit Child can also help you access and reclaim fragmented soul parts.

Develop a relationship with your Spirit Child and it will help you uncover the traumas that are at the root of destructive behavior patterns. A key to bring your dreams to reality, achieve emotional maturity and Radiant Health, the Spirit Child can bring to light the subtle and blatant traumas of childhood. Once acknowledged, the wound can be cleaned out and healed.

Trauma is often the foundation of limiting fear-based beliefs and dysfunctional behaviors, attitudes and perceptions. Healing trauma can dissolve negative imprints, eradicate feelings of insecurity and low self-esteem, eliminate dysfunctional, destructive, childish behaviors and actions and restore the natural flow of your creative energy, all of which supports greater conscious awareness and emotional growth and maturity. To identify, acknowledge and heal trauma is a cornerstone on *The Journey to Radiant Health*.

As an adult, the responsibility to heal is on you.

No one can do it for you.

The Spirit Child Can Access Buried Pain

The Spirit Child can provide you with simple answers and clear directions on how to heal your traumas. It is up to you to listen and act on its messages. Be aware that as a creative aspect of the emotional body, the Spirit Child's answers are not usually logical, but always are simple and make sense. Your Spirit Child will provide you with information, enabling you to reclaim your power and face your fears.

Contacting your Spirit Child will enable you to grow, change and heal. Ask your questions when you are fully ready, willing and prepared to hear and act on the Spirit Child's answers. Otherwise, the ego will rationalize the Spirit Child's answers as being nonsense. The ego will undermine your ability to clearly hear and trust the Spirit Child, and cause you to believe this Spirit Child stuff is just a bunch of mumbo-jumbo.

Because the information the Spirit Child provides will require you to look at your pain, the ego personality will react and resist. The ego does not want to explore old traumas. It does not care whether traumas fester or develop into dis-ease. The ego reacts to avoid pain, even if it means breaking destructive habits to become healthy. After treating your childhood traumas, the Spirit Child can take you on the next leg of *The Journey to Radiant Health*.

The Spirit Child Contains Your Dreams

You incarnated with your life purpose etched in your heart and mind. Your purpose was lightly veiled in the childhood dreams of who you wanted to be and what you wanted to do. Because of the parental, religious and cultural imprints that are experienced in childhood, those dreams can be lost. Deep in the recesses of your being, however, those dreams remain fresh and alive. The Spirit Child can access them. Developing a relationship with your Spirit Child will enable you to retrieve your dreams.

As you develop a relationship with your Spirit Child, ask it to reveal your childhood dreams. Write them down. The list might be as long as the things you like to do. It also might include things that you have long forgotten. Your Spirit Child will reveal the dreams and activities that inspire your passion, bring you joy and satisfaction and resonate with the deep knowledge of what you incarnated to accomplish.

Spirit Child Meditation

The Spirit Child meditation will introduce you to your Spirit Child. Read the meditation over thoroughly and then ask a friend to read it to you. Please follow the instructions and meditation precisely. Sit in a comfortable chair with your spine erect. Remove your shoes, watch and any jewelry. The meditation should take between 20 and 40 minutes to complete. Make sure you have ample time, in case it takes longer. Keep these three points in mind before starting:

- *Do not rush the meditation.*
- *Proceed slowly and take a deep breath between commands.*
- *Read the entire meditation to get a feel for the pace of it.*

1. Take three long, slow, deep breaths to release the tension from the day.

2. As you continue to breathe, begin to relax your body. Start with your feet. Relax your toes, feet and ankles. Relax your calves. Relax your knees. Relax your thighs. Breathe slowly and deeply.

3. Now relax your hips. Relax your stomach and lower back. Relax your chest and mid-back. Relax your upper back and shoulders. Relax your biceps and triceps. Relax your forearms. Relax your hands and fingers. Relax your neck and head. Relax your jaw. Relax your lips, mouth and tongue. Relax your eyes. Breathe deeply.
   Your entire body is fully relaxed.

4. Now visualize a curtain rising in front of you. See yourself in a meadow with rolling hills, green grass and a nearby stream. Listen to the gentle current of the water. See the beautiful green trees and the blue sky with scattered puffy clouds. Feel the sun warming your entire body.

5. Now, look straight ahead; a small figure is walking toward you. As it gets closer, you notice that it is a child. As the child walks towards you, notice its clothing. As the child gets closer, notice its face. Now as the child stands in front of you, look into its eyes. Notice the look on the child's face. Recognize the child is you.

   This is your Spirit Child.

6. Notice whether your Spirit Child looks happy, sad, angry or non-expressive. Ask her if there is anything that she needs. If your Spirit Child says yes, then listen carefully and tell her that you will do your best to fulfill her request.

7. Ask her if there is anything that she needs you to know. Listen closely to whatever she tells you. When she is finished speaking, acknowledge what she said. If you are unclear about what she said ask her for clarity. Do not make assumptions or try to interpret her words. Continue asking her questions until you are perfectly clear.

8. When she has nothing more to tell you, then ask her to give you a word. Only you and your Child will know this word. No one else is to ever know this word. Anytime your Spirit

Child needs your attention you will hear this word. Whenever you hear the word, you are to close your eyes and ask your Child what she needs. Now, ask your Spirit Child for the word.

9. After you receive the word, ask her if there is anything else that she needs to tell you. If she says yes, then listen carefully and respond. When she has nothing further to say, let her know that when she needs to contact you, she can just use the word, and no matter what you are doing you will come and see what she needs. Let her know that you will be here whenever she needs to talk with you.

10. When she is complete, take a deep breath and allow the picture to begin to fade. Reinforce the message that when she needs you, she can use the word and you will come. If she is not ready for you to go, ask her what else she needs to tell you. When she is finished, tell her that you will be right here, and all she needs to do is use the word and you will come right away.

11. Take a deep breath and come back to your body. Breathe deeply and feel yourself fully in your body. Take another deep breath and return your full awareness to the room; and when you are ready, you can open your eyes.

How to Maintain a Solid Relationship with Your Spirit Child

Whenever you hear the word that you received from your Spirit Child, it is important to close your eyes and ask her what she needs. Do not get caught in the ego trap of believing that you thought the word yourself, or that you are not hearing it. She is likely to use the word as soon as you have completed the meditation.

When you hear the word, find a quiet place and check in. If no quiet place is available, use a restroom for privacy; otherwise just close your eyes for a moment. If you are driving, pull to the side of the road and check in.

Your Spirit Child always has something important to say.

In the beginning, your Spirit Child is likely to use the word repeatedly, just to make sure that you will come when she calls. The more you respond the more that you will begin to trust the voice of Spirit. Be consistent and check in each and every time you hear the word. When doubting thoughts arise like "I must be making this up" or "I am not sure if I am really hearing the word," check in anyway.

When you hear the word, respond to it.

In the beginning, it is wise to check in with your Spirit Child three times a day: when you wake up in the morning, in the early afternoon and before you go to bed. Simply close your eyes, and trust that she will be there when you summon her. Ask your Spirit Child if she used the word. If she says yes, ask her why you did not hear it. Often she will let you know that you ignored the word, because you did not want to stop what you were doing or hear what she had to say, or you didn't believe that she was calling. When you know this to be the case, acknowledge your Spirit Child for being right. This will strengthen your bond of trust.

When Difficulties Arise in Reaching the Spirit Child

If you have trouble hearing or contacting your Spirit Child, be persistent in your efforts. Meditate daily with a clear intention to reach your Spirit Child. This will improve your ability to contact, hear and develop the trust and discrimination needed to follow the messages you receive. If you have contacted your Spirit Child and find that she does not respond to you, there could be a number of reasons. But they all boil down to one common denominator, a lack of trust.

Take an honest and introspective look at yourself to ascertain if you have trouble believing:

A. the Spirit Child is real or even exists.

B. the messages you have received.

These are not uncommon obstacles, and they can be overcome. Simply open your mind and your heart to the opportunity to heal. Also, if you experienced mental, physical or emotional abuse as a child, seeing your Spirit Child can rekindle those memories. The Spirit Child can represent a return to the original pain, trauma and suffering. This can make it very challenging to maintain contact with your Spirit Child.

Remember, the purpose is to heal, and to reclaim your dreams.

The Ego Can Disguise Itself As the Spirit Child

When the Spirit Child's messages are self-centered and self-serving, the ego is at work. If your Spirit Child is mean or filled with fear, it might be the ego. It can also be a representation or display of the actual feelings you felt but were not able to express during your childhood. The Spirit Child might also be mirroring the frustration you feel about not being able to trust your own instinct, intuition or heart-based feelings.

If you experience these or any other confusing scenarios, you might want to consider working with a holistic healthcare professional. There are many skilled professionals who can help. A list of holistic healthcare professionals can be found in Chapter 34.

Keeping a Clear Perspective on the Spirit Child

Contacting your Spirit Child is a step toward reaching the center of your emotional body, but the Spirit Child is a stepping stone to the Divine Child, not the Divine Child itself. Healing traumas, unraveling unhealthy imprints and belief systems brings you a step closer to emotional maturity and ego mastery. But keep in mind that developing a strong relationship with your Spirit Child is simply a precursor to reaching the emotional body's truth centers, the next layer in the emotional body and the next step on *The Journey to Radiant Health*.

-18-

The Truth Centers: Instinct, Intuition and Love

When you establish a trusting and committed relationship with your Spirit Child—which entails checking in every day, listening to its messages and following its directions—a magical event will take place. The relationship will reach harmonic resonance, the separation will dissolve and your Spirit Child will merge with you.

When integration occurs, you will be pulled into the truth centers.

The three truth centers, Instinct, Intuition and Love, occupy the third layer in the emotional body. They are Yin in nature and sit directly opposite the mental body's three constructive components: focus, commitment and discipline. When the Yin truth centers are used in concert with the Yang constructive components, the feminine and masculine energy is synthesized and bound to one another, creating the wholeness that enables you to access your Spirit, receive guidance from the Divine and commune with the Divine.

As a sentient being comprised of the energy of light, every cell in the body can be tuned to other fields of energy. The constructive components (see Chapter 28) can be used to attune your frequency to the truth centers and can greatly increase your vibration.

Higher vibrations resonate with the frequency of Love, and give birth to the Divine Child.

The Truth Centers: Another Sacred Trinity

The way the Sacred Trinity of Truth Centers works is fairly simple. The Ego, which resides at the gut, governs the masculine truth center—Instinct. This is the lowest truth center. The Soul, which resides at the Soul/solar plexus, governs the feminine truth center—Intuition. The Spirit, which resides in the heart, governs the Divine Child truth center—Love. This is the highest truth center.

Love is the center point of the Sacred Trinity of Truth Centers triangle. Love is born from the union of the masculine and component energy. The integration of the two brings you into the heart, which is where Love—which is the highest Truth one can put into Action—resides.

Each of the three truth centers also corresponds to a specific Chakra. A *Chakra* is defined as "a disk or wheel of energy." There are seven Chakras and each is located at a specific area that corresponds to the body. The Chakras are explored in detail in the Appendix.

The first four Chakras relate to the truth centers.

The Ego/gut–Instinct truth center accesses its information from the first and second Chakras. The Soul/solar plexus–Intuition truth center accesses its information from the third Chakra. The heart-Love center accesses its information from the fourth Chakra.

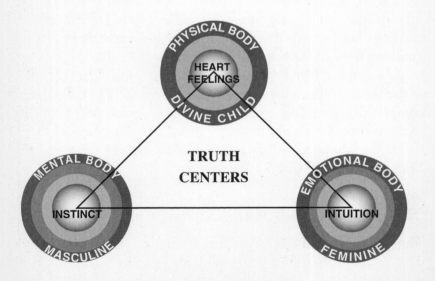

After establishing a relationship with your Spirit Child it becomes easier to access the truth centers. The truth centers, often described as a sixth sense or ESP—extra sensory perception—penetrate a stratum of non-ordinary reality and access a more profound source of information than ordinary, linear reality. The mental body gathers information from the external linear environment and processes it through the mind. The emotional body's truth centers, on the other hand, access information from the internal non-linear environment, including the Spirit realm, where it can be brought directly to the heart and put into action.

But that is not all.

The Truth Centers Translate
Subtle Frequencies into Information

The truth centers gather and process information in a way that is not available to the mental body. The mental body, linear in nature, is limited to the realms of logic, reason and tangible, scientific, provable forms of information. One has to transcend the mind in order to comprehend and explain the intangible, non-linear, mystical sources which convey the information accessed by the truth centers. It is nearly impossible to explain or understand decisions that are made based on one's feeling, inner knowingness, hunch or Divine guidance.

But that is what makes the truth centers unique.

The truth centers translate frequencies into information and are not dependent on logic, reason or scientific proof to validate their information. The truth centers operate in harmonic resonance with the subtle levels of consciousness, and the information from the heart truth center, in specific, comes from your Guides, Angels, Ascended Masters and Avatars.

The point is to develop your ability to listen to the heart, and follow its messages.

Information is energy, and all energy has a frequency. As stated in Chapter 1, Love produces a very high frequency. Consistent practice of conscious breathing brings you to a higher vibration, and when your vibration rises high enough, the information accessed is pure love, Agape.

It also is important to note that while the truth centers' information, especially the heart truth center, which sustains the frequency of Love, is always simple, it is not always easy to trust or act on. This is because the Ego often overrides the simple messages because it fears anything that arises from the unknown—that which does not arise from logic or reason.

Information from the higher realms is not linear or ruled by the same constraints and laws that apply to physical reality. The truth centers' information, which is fluid and flexible rather than rigid, straight and narrow, challenges you to practice the principles of Love and adapt, adjust and soften to life. Access the truth centers, especially the heart truth center, and you will find the simple answers to even the most complex questions.

THE EGO/GUT:
GOVERNOR OF INSTINCT

The Instinct truth center, governed by the Ego and masculine energy, is located in the lower abdominal region. Instinctive feelings are commonly associated with this area because "gut feelings," which are primarily energetic in nature, are felt in this section.

"Going with your gut" describes the strong, centered and grounded feeling that enables you to trust your instincts when confronted by a challenge, or attempting to solve a problem. Instinct is an ancient and primal sensory warning system. Its primary purpose is to alert you to imminent danger in your immediate external environment.

When it comes to Instinct, the most important thing to remember is that it is a reactive warning system. This is why Instinct ranks at the bottom of the Sacred Trinity of Truth Centers. While it can be an effective truth center, it can also be activated by fear, which is produced by the Ego. The Ego, being the governor of instinct, is the flaw that can make it undependable.

How Instinct Works

The Instinct truth center works by sensing the vibrations of the electro-magnetic fields, or frequency of energy, around you. Instinct detects the frequency of people with whom you come into direct contact, as well as those in your immediate proximity. It also detects the vibration in the places you enter or are about to enter.

Everything has its own frequency. Instinct detects the frequencies of people you meet, places you go and things around you like alleys, neighborhoods, animals and trees. Instinct deciphers frequency and translates the information into the language of sensation. The sensation produced by the frequency is what you feel in your gut.

The sensation is often described as a *"vibe," "sense"* or *"feeling"* you get about someone or something, such as: *"She has a mellow vibe," "I have a good sense about that place"* or *"I have a feeling that we should avoid that street."* Instinctive feelings like caution, apprehension, anxiety, comfort, relaxation or safety help you determine a course of action.

Come into contact with people or situations where a lower frequency—produced by dark thought forms and emotions—is in effect and your Instinct is activated, emitting a physiological sensation that causes you to be acutely aware of everything in your environment. The Instinct signal informs you that something is amiss even though there might be no ostensible reason to think so.

Fear, being the lowest frequency, can trigger the Instinct. Fear, which arises from the Ego, releases adrenaline into the body preparing it for fight or flight. While Instinct increases overall awareness, when triggered by fear, it actually decreases awareness. Fear causes Instinct to become muddled, causing confusion about what action to take or which direction to move. This can lead to emotional, mental and even physical paralysis.

Bombarding the senses with stimulus that constantly triggers instinctive reactions (like the excessive violence portrayed in the daily news and movies) can desensitize or overstimulate you. This can cause you to ignore Instinct's signals and warnings. To experience Radiant Health, limit the Ego from indulging in reaction-producing stimulus. This will enable you to maintain harmony with your Instinct, so that you will heed its signal to proceed with caution or stop before you are in imminent danger.

THE SOUL/SOLAR PLEXUS: GOVERNOR OF INTUITION

The Intuition truth center, governed by the Soul and feminine energy, is located at the solar plexus, just below the point where the ribs join on the front of the chest. Intuition is independent of the thought process and often contradicts logic, reason and common sense. Intuition is difficult to heed at times, because it can mean taking action contrary to what is expected.

When Intuition is followed, mysteriously and almost miraculously you will find yourself in the right place at the right time. It confers a sense of knowing, certainty, confidence and surety about your actions. This happens without external indicators or reasoning to validate the intuitive feelings that guide you. For example, a strong feeling to call your best friend suddenly washes over you, seemingly out of the blue. You follow it and discover that your friend needs help and wanted to call you, but was unable. This is Intuition at work.

Intuition, being a Yin/feminine element, does not resonate with the external environment, nor does it have a warning mechanism like the Yang/masculine Instinct. Intuition moves beyond the realm of the Ego and external environment to the inner realm of conscious awareness. It complements and balances your instinctual energy.

To access Intuition, turn your focus and attention inward. Let go of the thought process, meditate intently on the Soul/solar plexus and attune yourself with its subtle vibration. When an intuitive message becomes clear, you will feel pulled as if by a string to your destination. A well-developed Intuition enables you to attune to higher vibrations and access information from Saints, Sages or higher beings.

It is easy to judge the Intuitive feelings or messages that lead you to be in the right place at the right time as spooky, weird or coincidental. Unable to logically explain paranormal phenomena or unravel the mystery of Intuition, the mind dismisses the connections that arise from Intuition as a fluke or an accident. These explanations make the Ego feel safe and in control of its environment.

Trust Your Intuition

Learn to trust and follow your Intuition and you will experience a greater level of comfort and confidence in life. For example, trust and act on your Intuition to call a friend, and you will discover that he needs assistance. This is an empowering lesson in trusting your Intuition. Learning to trust your Intuition can be life changing because it enables you to take actions even though no tangible reason exists for doing so.

Intuition brings you into alignment with the creative universal process. Trust your Intuition and the need to know how you will arrive at an outcome and the need to control the process can be released. Rather than waiting for external signposts to validate or dictate your course of action, you will be more likely to *"go with the flow."*

People who always seem to be in the right place at the right time trust and follow their Intuition. They live in the moment, take risks and participate to the fullest extent in life. Every experience is an adventure and they make smooth transitions, flowing intuitively from one place to the next and from one set of circumstances to another. Rarely do they get upset or dwell on things that do not go their way because they have learned to trust the process of life. They know, intuitively, there is always a Divine reason for the events in life, even if the mystery does not reveal itself in the moment.

Learn to trust your Intuition and follow your heart, and you will not need to have all the answers or figure things out. Slow down, listen, and the answers will arise. Regardless of how well your Intuition is developed you might find that, at times, you disregard it. Keep in mind that you are working toward wholeness. A key to experiencing bliss rests in this realization. You can strive to be the best you can, but let go of the pressure to be perfect.

Intuition also can provide important information that can help restore health when you are ill. Meditate, and your Intuition can be used to uncover the contributing factors to your illness. It can also help you find people and remedies to help restore your health. Many remedies are available to treat many dis-eases, but only a few will be appropriate to you. Intuition is an avenue from which to turn your attention inward and check whether a specific protocol, remedy or treatment is appropriate for you.

Whenever your focus shifts from the internal to the external and you lose your direction and feel confused, return to conscious breathing and reconnect to the intuitive truth center. Regardless of what is going on in your external environment, the answers that will enable you to handle it effectively can be found by tapping into your inner guidance.

THE HEART:
GOVERNOR OF LOVE

The heart truth center, governed by Spirit and balanced between feminine and masculine energy, is located at the area of the physical heart. The heart merges Love and Truth into a perfect balance of feminine and masculine energy. The heart also harmonizes and integrates the Ego/gut–Instinct and the Soul/solar plexus–Intuition, as well as all feminine and masculine qualities. Love is born of the marriage between feminine and masculine.

As the heart integrates your masculine and feminine energies, you will feel healthy, balanced and creative. The heart captures the intensity of the feminine fire of Passion and the power of the masculine fire of Will, using them to support the expression of Love in a mindful, considerate, honorable and utterly exquisite manner.

By entering the heart, you can express the full power of Love.

The heart does not judge any emotion; it simply seeks to pour forth Love. This is the heart's Spiritual charge. It is the sacred container of Love and its supply of Love is unlimited. In the context of emotions, the Heart simply sees an opportunity to express them in an authentic, genuine and sincere manner. It is from the heart that the depth of your soul and feelings spring forth.

The heart accesses and expresses your true nature, Spirit.

Reclaim Your Spirit

Spirit cannot be contained, domesticated or civilized. Spirit is often feared and repressed because its expression is unconventional. Yet within Spirit is a wholesome beauty that experiences the sacred in all things and a wisdom that takes nothing for granted.

Because the heart does not judge, it views no emotion or expression as wrong. Attune to the heart and the full and immediate expression and release of pain or suffering will take place. The heart's truth will not suffocate emotion because protocols such as deadlines or being in mixed company deem it inappropriate. The heart's expression cannot be bound by rules and regulations. Love and truth as creative energy cannot always be packaged in a neat little container for the convenience of others.

The Heart Transcends the Three Rules
for Expressing Anger

In the chapter on anger three rules were set out for the healthy expression of anger. When you access the heart, however, there is no need for them. The heart, which expresses only Love, will take anger's energy, center it (determination to stand in the highest truth—Love) and use it to uncover the hidden pain, agony, hurt or despair, and express it in a Divine way. The heart knows that anger is nothing more than a protective energy that arises to hide the dashed expectations that lead to sadness. The heart knows that sadness and grief arise from the desire to express the pain of that which was loved and lost.

Expressing Your Heart's Love Facilitates Radiant Health

The heart's Love (see "Heart-Based Qualities of Agape," Chapter 19) needs to be expressed to experience Radiant Health. When you express the heart's Love, pain and suffering, anger and frustration, sadness and grief dissolve, stress and tension is eliminated and the risk of illness and dis-ease are dramatically reduced. Think, speak and act from the heart; this is the way to express your true nature, Spirit, and is also the road to Radiant Health.

Expressing your heart's Love provides others an environment of safety and comfort. A warm and open heart embodies and expresses loving qualities like forgiveness, acceptance, compassion and trust. These qualities enable you to express and release any pain and suffering, sorrow and grief that would otherwise burden your heart.

The Heart and the Ego

Putting Love into Action—step two on *The Journey to Radiant Health*—seats you in the heart's Love. Being seated in the heart's Love, the Ego cannot control you or cause harm to others. The heart's frequency, which resonates to Love, supersedes the Ego's frequency, which resonates to fear. When seated in the heart's vibration, it is easy to recognize Ego and dismiss its selfish desires. The heart dissolves the Ego through pure loving expressions like forgiveness and compassion. The heart fully embraces the Ego without the need to control, subdue, overrule or overpower it. Apply step two, Put Love into Action, and the Love in your heart will overcome all Ego uprisings.

Summation of How to Use the Truth Centers

Use the truth centers in ascending order. When Instinct alerts you to danger, return to conscious breathing. As conscious breathing raises your vibration, you will naturally ascend to the next truth center, Intuition. Listen for guidance and trust the direction you receive from your Intuition. Finally, ascend into the heart and carry out its Spiritual charge: Put Love and Truth into Action. When you enter the heart, its exalted qualities—Agape and Wisdom—will stream forth, enabling you to transcend the Ego and act with greater awareness and compassion.

The Emotional Body Center: Love and Agape

Practice step two, Put Love into Action, on *The Journey to Radiant Health,* and you are catapulted to the center of the emotional body. From the center of the emotional body, only Agape, the highest and purist form of love, is expressed. From the center of the emotional body every component in every layer of the emotional body falls into alignment with the expression of Agape, which is God, Love and Light itself.

Agape, unconditional love, glorifies the Divine, expressing itself through thirty-two distinct qualities (see the last page of this chapter). Each quality is important, yet four are distinguished as being essential to practice in every moment:

Forgiveness

Acceptance

Compassion

Trust

FACT is an acronym that will help you remember the four qualities.

Humanity as a whole, being entrenched in the darkness of ignorance for so many eons, has been slow to grasp the profound healing powers of *FACT*. Humankind has been even slower to embrace and perform them openly and with regularity. Spiritual masters epitomize *FACT*, and encourage, support and prescribe their daily use as a Spiritual tonic and discipline. As heart-based Spiritual qualities, *FACT* is capable of dissolving blockages of energy in the emotional, mental and physical bodies. They are also the perfect qualities to put into action to heal the wounds of the Spirit Child.

Put *FACT* into action, and healing takes place.

The Vibration of Agape

Agape emits the highest frequency in the universe. The conscious application of forgiveness, acceptance, compassion and trust—the four most important expressions of Agape—can melt away disharmony and suffering. When any quality of Agape is put into action with a sincere heart and a focused mind, it will keep your vibration as high as possible, and produce spontaneous, immediate healing.

The Foundation of *FACT*

The qualities of *FACT* are unlimited in their ability to transform dis-ease-producing thoughts, emotions and behaviors. Each quality will be discussed individually, which includes an exercise to help you put it into action. Listed below is the unique characteristic each quality possesses to reduce or eliminate a specific condition or dis-ease.

Forgiveness enables you to release judgments and anger.

Acceptance keeps you emotionally centered.

Compassion reduces or alleviates pain and suffering.

Trust transcends fear by affirming that all things are in Divine order.

The ego, its behaviors and components of separation, make it hard to practice *FACT*. A complete list of ego behaviors can be found in Chapter 26, and its components of separation in Chapter 27. Be unyielding in your efforts to practice step two, Put Love into Action, and *FACT* will eliminate ego behaviors and dis-ease-producing emotions.

FORGIVENESS

The practice of forgiveness is not easy, but is essential on *The Journey to Radiant Health*. Forgiveness is the only true healing remedy that can alleviate anger-based emotions (which are directed outward towards others) such as resentment, hatred, irritation, bitterness and frustration; and sadness-based emotions (which are directed inward towards the self) such as guilt, shame, hopelessness and despair. Ego behaviors such as blame, judgment, criticism, condemnation and unfulfilled expectations can also be healed by the act of forgiveness. Emotional, mental or physical abuse such as discrimination, betrayal, racism, infidelity, assault, rape or murder are transgressions that cannot be healed by anything other than forgiveness.

Left unchecked, all of the previously mentioned emotions and behaviors lead to dis-ease.

To forgive requires a number of clear actions. The actions have little to do with the transgressor and more to do with transforming your attitude. Because of this, the actions that lead to forgiveness can be challenging, confrontive and even painful. But when they are completed, they ensure that your forgiveness has been established on a solid foundation.

The Requisites of Forgiveness

Often, the pain and suffering caused by a transgression or injustice are so intense and have such long-lasting ramifications that resentments, anger, hatred and the desire for revenge can be justified as being righteous, expected and even acceptable. This makes taking the high road of forgiveness a far more challenging venture.

Fortitude, leadership, courage, integrity, dignity, humility and the ability to detach are qualities needed to successfully walk the path of forgiveness. But there is one quality that is absolutely essential to practice forgiveness, an open heart. Opening your heart to forgive can, quite possibly, be the most challenging requirement of all. This is especially true when you have been the victim of cruel and malicious actions. But to regain your peace of mind and emotional center you have to fully forgive. This means that your anger must be transmuted and channeled into motivation and determination to stand in the highest truth, Love. Only then will you be able to feel your pain, share your grief, shed your tears and release whatever emotional charge (desire for revenge, justice, etc.) that you have towards the transgressor. When you have done all of this, you will be able to face the transgressor without feeling any emotional charge.

Only then can you say that you have truly extended the hand of forgiveness.

To open your heart, you must be willing to forgive. To do this you will need to ask yourself some tough questions. For example, *"What is causing me to choose to hold onto my anger, resentment and frustration?" "How is my reluctance to forgive affecting my emotional, mental and physical health and well-being?" "What benefits do I expect to get from holding a resentment towards the person who hurt me?"*

When you can answer these questions, you will get a clearer understanding of how your anger, resentments and desire for vengeance are affecting you. The answers are what you need to release in order to put yourself in a position to forgive.

You cannot truly forgive until you let go.

Forgiving Others Heals You

The intensity of the pain and suffering you experience in relation to a transgression or injustice is in direct proportion to your defiance, resistance or reluctance to forgive. On the other hand, when you forgive others, you become the main beneficiary of the forgiveness. Because the moment you forgive, all the resentment, anger, hatred and vengeance carried in your heart dissolves.

In Alcoholics Anonymous, it is said, *"Carrying a resentment is like drinking poison and expecting the other person to die."* Forgiveness detoxifies the poisons of anger, resentment and the desire for revenge and restores emotional, mental and, in some cases, even physical health and well-being.

Love starts at home.

Home is where your heart is.

By first forgiving yourself, it becomes easier to forgive others. This means releasing self-judgment and blame. The more you forgive yourself, the more capable you will be of forgiving others. The peace and serenity that you experience as you forgive will inspire you to continue to practice forgiveness.

The Meaning of Sin, and the Power in Forgiving It

Offenses that need to be forgiven are commonly labeled *sins*. In Spanish the word *sin* means "without," and a sin simply describes an action performed without love. Sin is synonymous with ego because any action that arises from the ego is without love. When a sin is committed, the greatest challenge is to suspend judgment and provide the missing love, by bestowing forgiveness.

Loveless ego actions produce a low frequency and will magnetically attract the same low frequency in return. This is called Karma —the law of cause and effect. Ego actions, therefore, do not need to be avenged; the law of Karma will eventually balance all injustices.

On the other hand, when you respond to a low-frequency ego action with a high-frequency quality like forgiveness, you will sidestep the lower frequency. This simply means that by forgiving, you will not get into an argument, feel angry or judge the other person. Protect yourself with the higher frequency of forgiveness and disease-producing emotions and behaviors such as anger, blame, judgment, condemnation, cynicism, resentment and hatred will fall by the wayside.

Forgiveness in Action

The path of forgiveness is one of fortitude, character, vision and inspiration. The following stories are exceptional examples of forgiveness in action.

The first occurred after the 1992 uprisings in Los Angeles, California. Reginald Denny, a truck driver, was brutally beaten during the turmoil. He did nothing to provoke the attack; he was simply in the wrong place at the wrong time. Public sentiment clearly favored condemnation of his attackers. But, Denny would not cave in to public sentiment. When the men who battered him stood trial for their actions, Denny openly spoke with them and dialogued with the young men's relatives. When Denny spoke to the media he extended the hand of forgiveness, and his tone was one of understanding.

Denny's act of forgiveness was courageous and inspirational.

The second involves basketball legend Michael Jordan, whose father was murdered, the victim of a car-jacking perpetrated by two youths. The excruciating pain and suffering caused by this senseless act of violence would sorely test even the most openhearted person to practice forgiveness. Michael, however, went beyond the call to simply forgive. He actually met with the two young men before they stood trial and, in a press conference held after his meeting, Michael publicly expressed forgiveness.

Michael Jordan displayed the fortitude and courage to forgive.

Below are two forgiveness exercises. The first will help you forgive yourself for anything you might have done to harm yourself or another. The second will help you release anger and forgive others for their transgressions towards you.

FORGIVENESS EXERCISES
Exercise A. Forgiving Yourself

1. Write down some things you have done that still cause you to feel shame, guilt, embarrassment or regret.

2. Pray for the ability to forgive yourself.

3. Look into a mirror, focus on conscious breathing, maintain contact with your eyes and, using your name, say "____, I love and forgive you." When you can recall the action without feeling pain, guilt, shame or any other emotions, you are complete.

4. When disparaging or judgmental thoughts or emotions arise about you or others, immediately let go of them. Say to the arising thoughts or emotions, *"You are completely forgiven, so leave me entirely alone."*

Exercise B. Forgiving Others

1. Think of someone you feel angry or resentful towards.

2. Pray to release your resentment, anger or hatred.

3. Think of every good thing that you want for your life, and as you pray to forgive that person, also pray that he/she receives every good thing that you want.

4. Meditate on the vision of putting your hand on his/her heart and forgiving. Do not stop until you feel love pouring forth from your heart into his/her heart.

5. If the anger or resentment resurfaces, repeat steps 1, 2 and 3 as necessary until the resentment is dissolved. When you feel peaceful when thinking about the individual, you have forgiven.

6. Take immediate action anytime you feel anger. Forgive the person before the anger turns into a judgment or resentment and permeates your consciousness.

ACCEPTANCE

Challenges and obstacles are a natural part of life. They do not always arise in relationship to your actions. Nor are they always a sign that something is wrong. When challenges and obstacles arise, they give you a chance to slow down and reevaluate your decisions and actions. The practice of acceptance is the first step towards admitting that life is filled with things that are beyond your ability to control or change. Floods, hurricanes, earthquakes, the economy, traffic jams, other people's words and actions, and even your race, color and age are just a few examples. Included in the list are also the times when you will experience intense feelings and react, saying or doing something that you will wish you had not.

You can try to control and influence other people and events, and when you are successful you will feel excited. But when you are not, you will feel irritated, frustrated, disappointed or resentful. Either way, trying to control or influence others and/or events is a gamble that will always put you on a roller coaster of emotional highs and lows.

Whatever form they take, challenges and obstacles make one thing clear: the only power you possess is the power to change your attitudes, perceptions and beliefs. Maintain an attitude of acceptance and you free yourself from reacting. Acceptance reduces stress and tension, lowers your blood pressure and keeps you mentally clear and emotionally centered. Practicing acceptance enables you to direct your attention towards finding solutions rather than wasting time worrying about problems.

You can restrain your words, moderate your actions, detach from your thoughts, strengthen your character, open your heart and change your attitudes and perceptions because you always have the power to change yourself.

This is the impetus for practicing acceptance.

The Power of Acceptance

Practicing acceptance empowers you to acknowledge your errors, amend your actions and behaviors, release self-judgment and criticism, pardon the oversights of others, and go with the flow rather than struggle. Practicing acceptance enables you to put your efforts and energy towards changing yourself, trusting in a higher power and adapting to your environment. Acceptance eliminates the need to control.

Acceptance enables you to handle obstacles with grace and poise. Self-acceptance makes it easier to admit, share and display the pain, hurt, disappointment and vulnerability that arise when sudden and tragic events prove that you are not in control.

Acceptance Heals Dis-eased Emotions and Behaviors

Acceptance is the antidote for impatience.

It can also ameliorate or completely neutralize other dis-eased emotions including frustration, irritation, anxiety, agitation, disappointment, helplessness, despair, worry, fear and regret. Practicing acceptance can help you manage emotional reactions, and ego behaviors such as competition, resistance or struggle. Practicing acceptance keeps your creative energy flowing freely, making it unlikely that dis-eased emotions or behaviors will exist long enough to metamorphose into a physical dis-ease.

One mark of emotional maturity is being able to maintain your balance and integrity when life's unforeseen events throw your well-conceived plans into disarray. Acceptance helps you to do this. It keeps you emotionally centered and even-tempered, and mentally clear and focused when everything around you is chaotic.

An attitude of acceptance enables you to embrace pain or tragedy in the same way you embrace joy and happiness.

Acceptance is akin to surrender. But unlike the negative connotations associated with surrender, acceptance does not mean giving up, abandoning your dreams or settling for less. To accept simply means to be able to let go of the need to fight, struggle, resist or use force to get your way.

Acceptance keeps you relaxed and serene.

Self-Acceptance

In post-modern society, self-worth and self-acceptance have increasingly become determined by material acquisition and wealth, charm and charisma, and physical appearance.

Manipulated by the commercial media from the time one is old enough to read or watch TV, the general population is spoon-fed a steady diet of competition-based consumerism. The dictates of competitive consumerism are to target specific individuals and segments of society such as children, teenagers, adults, the elderly, and ethnic and religious groups. Emotionally manipulative messages are developed to convince the targeted audience that the products they are buying will improve their self-worth and cause them to enjoy greater acceptance among their peers.

It is challenging to remain unaffected by these messages.

Commercial-consumer messages have saturated every area of daily life. On the TV, radio, internet, newspapers, billboards and magazines, they mandate what kind of job you need to have, how you need to look and the things you need to obtain to be viewed as sexy, successful and popular.

It is important to practice self-acceptance because commercial messages do not dare mention your Divine beauty and inherent perfection.

Practice self-acceptance and you can break free from consumer commercialism, stand on your own and release the need to be like the crowd. Self-acceptance enables you to affirm your uniqueness and step away from self-judgment and self-criticism.

Gratitude: The Cousin of Acceptance

Cultivating an attitude of gratitude begins by owning that you have the power to change. This power enables you to accept who you are, what you have, and the things that you cannot control. You always have the choice of how to perceive the events of your life. Dolly Parton says that instead of counting sheep when she goes to bed, she counts her blessings. To cultivate an attitude of gratitude, make it a habit to focus on your blessings rather than the tragedies.

The more you accept, the more gratitude you will cultivate, the more peace you will feel and the more beauty you will experience. An attitude of gratitude instills feelings of equanimity, harmony and happiness. Glean the positive from the hand that life deals to you and you will experience peace of mind and remain firmly rooted in the power of love.

The self-acceptance exercise below was designed to help you let go of who or what you believe you should be and accept yourself as you are. Because self-acceptance calls for self-love, the exercise can be challenging. If the exercise is difficult, be gentle, find and honor your own pace. Repeat the exercise as often as you can. The second exercise can help you release resistance, struggle, impatience or frustration.

EXERCISE A: SELF-ACCEPTANCE

1. Stand in front of a mirror, make eye contact, breathe deeply and proclaim sincerely with all your heart, *"I love you just as you are,"* five times.

2. Maintain your eye contact and proclaim with all your heart, *"You are Divine and God loves you,"* five times.

3. Repeat phrases #1 and #2, five times when you wake up in the morning and before you go to bed.

EXERCISE B: ACCEPTANCE

When something that is beyond your ability to change—a situation, person or condition—causes you to feel irritated, anxious or fearful, put the following steps into action.

1. Return to conscious breathing. Remain conscious of the breath until the mind becomes still and the energy of the emotions dissipate.

2. Pray for the strength to accept the person or situation. Turn your focus and attention inward, shifting your energy away from the situation and towards yourself.

3. Change your attitude. View the person or situation as an instrument that enables you to practice acceptance.

4. Cultivate an *"Attitude of Gratitude."* Find something positive about the situation, condition or person, even if the best you can do is to simply acknowledge that you have been given an opportunity to develop and strengthen your character and ability to practice acceptance.

5. Practice acceptance regularly. View every person, encounter, situation or condition as an opportunity to become aware of negative thoughts or distressing emotions, and to shift them by returning to conscious breathing and putting the practice of acceptance into that action.

COMPASSION

As is true with each Spiritual quality found in the center of the emotional body, compassion requires an open heart. To demonstrate compassion is to look plainly at pain and suffering and seek to reduce or alleviate it. To personify compassion is to look beyond superficial differences, suspend judgment and criticism, provide reassurance and empathize with others and see them as yourself.

A compassionate attitude embodies the Spiritual qualities of wisdom, patience, sincerity, kindness, tolerance, consideration, forgiveness, acceptance and trust. Being compassionate is to be fully present, aware and mindful to listen and act with an open heart. Doing this will enable you to comfort those who are afraid, in pain, grieving, or who otherwise demonstrate a need for understanding and healing.

Compassion Is the Higher Octave of Forgiveness

Forgiveness alleviates the suffering caused by anger, releases its emotional charge and moves you to its higher octave, compassion. Anger's emotional charge is what keeps you from being able to perceive the pain in the person that hurts you or those you love. After the emotional charge dissolves, you gain a new perspective and can perceive the deeper pain that caused him to strike out. Now, you are ready to move to put compassion into action.

Compassion Can Alleviate the Suffering Caused by Anger

Remember that anger is a common mask that is used to hide various forms of pain and suffering including sadness or grief, hurt or disappointment, and despair or hopelessness. Keep this in mind when you are in the presence of one who is angry and you will be able to see their pain. This is why it is essential to forgive acts of anger that have been directed towards you or someone you love. Forgiveness enables you to experience healing and then provide compassion.

Those who are angriest receive great benefit from the healing power of compassion. When someone is expressing anger in any of its unhealthy forms, including rage or depression, they do not feel safe enough to express the underlying pain.

A safe outlet is needed to transform the energy of anger from destructive to constructive. When you open your heart without judgment and listen with compassion, you empower a healthy expression of the anger. Your compassion can help transform the angry energy from destructive to constructive. By being a vessel of compassion—listening with sincerity and empathy—the emotional charge of the anger can be released.

When the emotional charge linked to the anger dissipates, the hidden pain can rise to the surface.

Compassionate Listening

To listen with compassion is to be mindful to hold your tongue, temper your thoughts, and support and empower others to identify and acknowledge their pain. The safety you provide by being a compassionate listener enables others to unmask their pain and come to their own conclusions about how to heal it. Surrendering what you think or believe would best serve them creates a compassionate space that supports the unfolding of their process. Listening with compassion also enables you to let your words be guided and inspired by the Divine.

Soothing and kind words, a quiet countenance, a soft and supportive glance, a gentle smile, a loving gesture and an open heart and mind also are expressions of compassion. A compassionate heart nurtures, listens with sincerity and responds when asked.

Those who have experienced a loss such as a child, parent, good friend, sibling or lover need and deserve compassion. So do those who are battling a life-threatening illness, have lost their job or home or are single parents struggling to raise kids. But the plain Jane and Joe that work a nine to five job or serve the community also need compassion.

To be compassionate with others, you must first be compassionate with yourself.

Being compassionate with yourself enhances your ability to have compassion for others. As you heal the split between your masculine and feminine energy, the mind and heart are reunified. A balanced heart-mind approach is born as the feminine creative-intuitive energies merge with the masculine structured-discipline energies. This balance enables you to step away from the hard-line masculine, "pull yourself up by the bootstraps" mentality. Equality between the heart and mind enables you to bring forth compassionate actions that help restore health and well-being.

The Indian Avatar Sathya Sai Baba says, "To the hungry love is food, to the thirsty love is water, to the naked love is clothing, and to the cold love is shelter."[1] Expressing compassion is marked by your ability to recognize and offer the most appropriate form of love in the moment it is needed. The simplicity inherent in compassion moves to ease pain and suffering.

Regardless of the form that love takes—whether it is food, shelter, clothing, listening or cheerfulness—the compassion with which it is given will be felt by those who receive it.

The Spiritual leader of the Tibetan people, the Dalai Lama, said, "Compassion is a peaceful, gentle and powerful force that helps us develop the very qualities we need to attain our goal of happiness."[2] As you display compassion by your actions, the needs of others will be satisfied and your feelings of happiness and well-being will be amplified. The exercise below will help you put compassion into action.

COMPASSION EXERCISE

1. Pick five people whose actions cause you to feel irritation, impatience or some other form of anger. They can be friends, acquaintances or people you pass on the street.

2. Look beyond their superficial actions and find the underlying pain or suffering.

3. Pray for the healing of their emotional, mental and physical bodies.

4. Pick one person out of the five and pray for guidance to find actions that will help alleviate the suffering.

5. Put the guidance you receive into action.

TRUST

Because trust is the one component that can allay your fears of the unknown, it is arguably the most essential as well as the most powerful element among the four essential qualities of Agape. Just as compassion is a higher octave of forgiveness, trust is a higher octave of acceptance.

Trust and faith are often used interchangeably. However, faith is only needed once in a person's life. Faith is essential the first time you experience a situation in which only God's direct intervention can rescue you. At that moment you step out onto the ledge of action and leap from the cliff of faith into the valley below with nothing but the parachute of God's grace to save you.

One of two things will happen:

You die, in which case you never need to have faith again.

Or, you survive, in which case you never need to have faith again.

When you survive, however, you have had a direct experience in which the Divine has taken care of you. Now, you can build on that experience, and every time you are faced with an impossible situation or task, you can *trust* that you will be okay. Trust in God makes this possible.

Trust enables you to transcend the nature of acceptance, in order to flow with the mystery of life and walk the Spiritual path with confidence, grounded in the wisdom that everything is in Divine order. Trust enables you to put love into action during the most trying moments on *The Journey to Radiant Health,* with the knowledge that you do not have to have all the answers.

While the phrase *"Everything happens for a reason"* flows easily from the lips, an unexplainable event will often put your ability to trust to the test. Although there is a purpose for your life and everything that happens in it, moments will arise when there will not be an easy answer to the question, *"Why?"* The reasons behind mysterious events such as the sudden, accidental death of a loved one or the bad things that happen to people are often unclear and seemingly beyond comprehension. The mind can search for logical explanations, but often, none exist. Without the trust that everything is in Divine order, the ego will conjure up some far-fetched reason to help you feel more secure and in control.

Trust quiets the mind, counteracts the fear, anger or confusion that accompanies unexplainable events and enables you to honor the mystery of life. When you trust that the Creator loves you and everyone and everything else equally, you can maintain an open heart and act from a loving higher state of consciousness.

Trust Enables You to Move beyond Illusion

One acronym for fear is: *False Evidence Appearing Real.* Fear is a product of the ego, and duality is a physical illustration of false evidence appearing real. There is no reality in separation; this is an illusion caused by the belief that duality is reality. But when the mind asserts the illusion that duality is reality, it enables the ego to reinforce the concept of separation.

Trust your heart and be guided by common sense and you will overcome the ego concept of separation. For example, while your fingers are separate from your toes, your body connects them to one another. In the same way, you are a unique entity, apparently distinct and separate from your friends and family. But you are connected to everyone and everything else in existence. Trust the information brought forth from your truth centers and your connection to all things will become apparent.

Overcoming Fear through Trust

It is easy to get caught up in fear, especially when you are faced with the unknown. For example, fear and doubt can sabotage your peace and serenity when you lose your job and do not know where the money to pay the rent will come from.

Unless you counteract the fear by trusting and taking action, you will likely magnetically attract to you that which you fear. So when you feel afraid, shift your attention away from the fear and return to conscious breathing. Confirm that you are a child of God, pray to God for assistance and trust that help is on the way. Then engage in loving actions. For example, call your friends and family and ask them for job leads, pick up the newspaper or get on the internet and do some searching. Make as many contacts as you can and let everyone know that you would appreciate any help that they have to offer.

After you have taken every action you can think of, sit quietly in meditation and reaffirm that you are safe and that you are always connected to Spirit. Place your trust in the Divine, keep your heart open and know that everything is in perfect order. Confirm that you have everything you need right here in this moment, and trust that when you need something it will appear at the exact moment that you need it.

Trust the Teachings of the Masters

When you cannot muster up enough trust to affirm that you are fully loved and that everything will be okay, pick up any Spiritual text that you can find and begin reading. You can read the Bible, the Bhagavad Gita, the Tao Te Ching, Buddha's teachings, or Spiritual texts such as *The Course in Miracles*. You can also read the writings of masters such as Sathya Sai Baba or Paramahansa Yogananda. Reading Spiritual texts will infuse your mind with higher vibrations, rekindle your trust in the Divine order of things and inspire you to act from the heart.

The masters exemplified love in their own unique ways and left us with great teachings to inspire us on this human journey. Buddha taught the Four Noble Truths and the Noble Eight-Fold Path as a way to end suffering. Lao Tzu taught the nature of the Tao and how to move in harmony with the ebb and flow of life. Jesus taught the New Covenant which is to love God with all your heart, mind and soul, and to love one another the same way. Gandhi taught the path of non-violent struggle and how to overcome adversity with love and devotion.

Each of these masters was a living model of trust in action. They listened to their heart, accessed the storehouse of universal knowledge contained within it and acted on what they received. By modeling trust in action and following the heart, every master leaves a powerful legacy.

You can be a master too. At the root of every master's teachings is the message to open your heart, be guided by the principles of love and trust the Divine order in all things. When you follow this formula you can be confident in your actions and you will leave a legacy of being a person who put love into action.

Trust Your Heart

By trusting your heart, you can live as an example of love. When you put love into action, ethics, morals and laws will become obsolete. Love transcends morals and ethics because love envelops them. Taoists claim that the need to have a code of morals and ethics merely demonstrates that we no longer trust the basic goodness that exists in our own heart. When the love in our heart is lost, we turn to defining concepts of right and wrong, and good and bad.

Dualistic concepts such as right and wrong or good and bad trap you into the limitations of acting from the ego. They force you to rely on external manmade laws rather than trusting the goodness in your heart. They also can cause you to look outside of yourself for knowledge and answers. Know that you can access and model goodness at any moment in time by trusting your heart and following the principles of love.

When you make the decision to express love in thought, emotion and action, you actively engage in the process of trusting your heart. Take loving actions and although you may not see the fruit of your actions immediately, in the end love will prevail.

TRUST EXERCISE

1. When you are faced with a problem that is beyond your control, influence or ability to change, practice acceptance and pray to the Divine for guidance.

2. Open your heart and trust that you will receive a loving answer in the form of a loving action to carry out.

3. Patiently await and know that a loving answer will come. Do not act until you receive, with clarity and certainty, a loving answer.

4. When the answer arises from your heart, and resonates with the vibrations of love, take action. Be confident in the knowl-

edge that whatever the outcome, it will be for the highest good.

AGAPE

Agape is the golden thread that binds the Spiritual qualities of forgiveness, acceptance, compassion and trust. During the last two thousand years, humanity has been blessed by Spiritual masters and conscious leaders who left blueprints on how to put love in action. Their lives modeled the Spiritual qualities of *FACT* as they expressed love and truth in action.

For example, the master Buddha displayed the power of Agape by relinquishing his nobility to pursue the path of enlightenment. He freely sacrificed his comforts, security, right to his future position as king and his worldly possessions and riches. With great compassion, Buddha dedicated his life to instructing others on how to put an end to suffering. The path of asceticism he followed inspired many of his followers to seek and eventually find true inner peace and harmony. In exemplifying Agape, by carrying out his selfless acts with compassion, humanity was enriched.

The master Jesus demonstrated the power of Agape by trusting and forgiving. Jesus knew his ultimate fate, but never asked that it be changed. He walked the path in full knowledge that God loved him. Jesus performed charitable acts of healing, showing great care and concern for others while always keeping his focus and attention on the Lord. Jesus, by openly forgiving those who decreed his crucifixion and those who supported it, modeled Agape even as he was put to death.

Mahatma Gandhi and Martin Luther King Jr. displayed the power of Agape by being disciples of non-violence. By never wavering in their discipline and commitment to stand on the Spiritual ideal of Agape, in either word or deed, each became an example of Agape's quality of acceptance. By being living examples of acceptance, each man was able to display heart-based qualities such as self-sacrifice, courage, humility, perseverance and patience. By practicing acceptance and staying the course, they changed the course of a nation and a people, respectively.

Use the Heart-Based Qualities to Express Agape

FACT are four of the most powerful heart-based qualities that can be expressed by human beings. But by no means do they express the totality of Agape. Therefore, the emotional body chapter concludes with a list of the eighteen preeminent heart-based qualities of Agape. Directly underneath the qualities of Agape are the ten heart-based characteristics that will enhance your ability to express Agape. Keep your focus and attention on the heart; choose one quality to demonstrate each day, and by constant practice and being aware, in time they will mature into habit.

THE HEART-BASED QUALITIES OF AGAPE

Purity of Emotions Harmlessness

Non-violence Fearlessness

Cleanliness Detachment

Equanimity Steadiness

Humility Sacrifice

Study Charity

Patience Courage

Integrity Sympathy

Asceticism Inner Peace

Sweetness and softness of speech

Absence of greed and selfishness

Absence of mental fluctuation

Refraining from gossip

Control of the senses

Fortitude in disasters

Straightforwardness

Awareness of creation's unity

Absence of anger or resentment

Restraint from unrighteous acts

Only one road leads
to lasting peace and happiness:
the road of love

and the road of love
originates in the heart.

SECTION FIVE

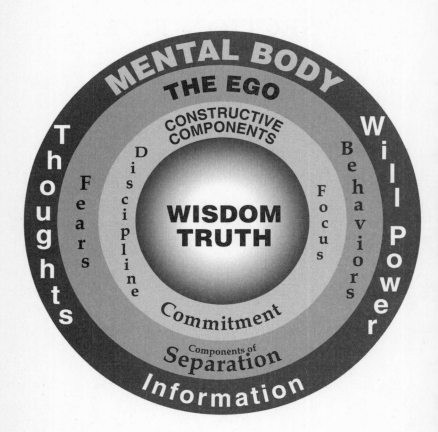

Color chart available at:
www.radiantkeys.com

20

The Mental Body

We are what we think.
All that we are arises with our thoughts.
With our thoughts we make the world.
Speak or act with a pure mind
and happiness will follow you as your shadow,
unshakable.
—The Dhammapada

The mental body represents the masculine energy in the Sacred Trinity. It sits to the right of the emotional body as its equal and harmonizing counterpart, as masculine energy rules the right side of the body. Mental body energy is linear and a straight line symbolizes its pattern of movement.

The primary function of mental/masculine energy is to provide structure to the creative energy of the emotional body. Unparalleled in its ability to bring form to the creative emotional body energy, the mind is the element most responsible for precipitating health, or its antithesis, dis-ease.

The mind's power can effect miraculous healings where no medicine or medical cure is administered. *Miracle* is the word used to describe the spontaneous healings that result from bringing pro-active mental energies such as commitment, focus or discipline into harmony with, and in support of, positive, healthy, creative emotional components such as attitudes, passion, imagination, perceptions and belief systems.

But, when unhealthy belief systems become rooted in unhealthy thought forms, attitudes and perceptions, the mind's power can lead to a breakdown in health. How you interpret your personal experiences greatly influences your degree of health. Fortunately, unhealthy belief systems, as well as unhealthy thoughts, attitudes and perceptions, can be changed.

The Dualistic Nature of the Mental Body

Mental body energy is like a double-edged sword.

On one hand, its power to generate immediate and even miraculous results is unlimited. Because it contains a number of components that can be used to increase awareness and dissolve blockages of energy, the mental body can facilitate healing and promote greater health.

In this way, the mental body is a powerful tool for health and well-being.

But the mental body also is home to the ego, the component responsible for the perception of separation and the causation of dis-ease. The ego represses and denies emotions and disrupts the free flow of creative emotional body energy. It is responsible for the majority of emotional, mental and physical dis-ease.

The ego can destroy health and cause suffering.

The Root Cause of Dis-ease

From a holistic viewpoint, all dis-ease is caused by blocked energy, and blocked energy results from resistance. Although resistance can arise in context to any number of things, it has two common denominators.

1. Resistance originates in the mental body and arises from fear. Whenever fear, in any of its manifold forms, is experienced and consequently repressed or denied by the ego, it becomes lodged in the emotional body. This ego action blocks the free flow of creative emotional energy.

2. The roots of resistance can be traced to one of the three bodies' basic functions: feeling or expressing emotions, opening the mind

to new thoughts or ideas, or taking action. When the fear that has caused the resistance is not uncovered and resolved, it will manifest as dis-ease at some point in time. In the physical body, it will show up by accidents (although you know that there are no real accidents—see Chapter 10), injuries or illness. In the mental body, it will manifest as obsessions, confusion or insanity. In the emotional body, it will be expressed by unmanageable emotional states such as rage or depression.

The Root of Radiant Health

Consistently, research indicates a correlation between thoughts and emotions on the one hand and physical health on the other. This information is causing the conventional Western medical model to rethink its ideology and beliefs concerning the role and application of medicine and the origin of dis-ease.

This paradigm, new to the West, is not really new at all.

Ancient wisdom has always asserted that dis-ease does not necessarily start in the physical body, nor is dis-ease limited to it. Furthermore, all holistic/alternative healing arts owe their longevity to a strict adherence to the axiom that healing starts in the mind and addresses the whole being, not just the body.

Commit to unearth the root cause of dis-ease and you will experience a greater degree of healing.

The three mental body constructive components—focus, commitment and discipline—play an important part in changing core thoughts and beliefs from unhealthy to healthy. The three will be studied in detail later, but for now it will suffice to say that putting the constructive components into action is the catalyst that can shift fear to love, separation to wholeness, helplessness to empowerment and dis-ease to health. Without the healthy mental body components, the desired effect—integration—will not take place. Further, if integration does not become a primary consideration, any attempts at healing will be inadequate and short-lived.

The Mental Body's Outer Layer

The mental body has its own place of importance in helping to restore balance between your masculine and feminine energy. The three fundamental mental body components—Thoughts, Information and Will—can be used proactively to affect your life. Complementary exercises follow the description of each component in the next chapter. Each exercise has been designed to increase your awareness and inspire healthy changes in your life.

21

Thought Forms

Thought forms are seeds of energy that can have a profound effect on your life. When ample time, focus and attention is given to a specific thought form, its energetic seed will sprout and manifest into physical reality. The energy contained in thought forms can be used to spontaneously shift your present reality.

Thoughts are cause, and what they produce are effects.

For example, many individuals can bend a metal spoon or fork simply by focusing their thought form energy. Focusing on the thought to bend the fork or spoon eventually produces the desired effect. The energy from the thought form causes the spoon or fork to bend as if it were made of rubber. The thought form energy is the cause, and the bending utensil is the effect.

When thoughts of love are sown, love is reaped.

When thoughts of fear are sown, fear is reaped.

How Thought Forms Manifest into Physical Form

Thought form energy arises from the mind and is carried into the ethers. The energy from an aimless or unfocused thought seed carries a short distance, dissipating before a distinct manifestation can take place. A clear-intentioned and well-focused seed of thought carries its energy much farther, crystallizing and manifesting in physical form. The instant materialization of thought form's energy is commonly referred to as a miracle.

Hence the adage: *Be careful of what you pray for, you might get it!*

Integrating the feminine component of Passion with the masculine component of Will can germinate the thought form seed. Passion and Will intensify the thought form energy, enabling it to grow stronger and manifest fruit quicker. The Divine Child component, Action, further stabilizes the thought form energy, ensuring its crystallization and eventual materialization.

Thought Form Energy Transference

Like a radio wave, thought forms transmit a wide range of frequencies. The range covers every frequency from the lowest, fear, to the highest, love. Thought forms can be transmitted from one individual to another, and can be tuned in or out, or changed. When you find yourself thinking about something unpleasant or disturbing, you can tune your thoughts to a higher frequency.

A common thought form energy transference pattern occurs through simple communication or interaction. Take a person who is upset, for example. Although his/her distress has nothing to do with you, during the course of telling you about the problem, you might find yourself feeling upset.

What has occurred is thought form energy transference.

A subtler example of thought form energy transference can take place when you are in the presence of a disturbed individual. Although you might not personally interact with him, you might begin to feel agitated, anxious or upset. When this happens, the vibrations of his thought forms are affecting you.

Being unaware or not believing in the phenomenon of thought form energy transference does not negate its power or make you immune to its effects. To keep from being affected by thought form energy transference, you can engage in higher vibration thought forms that focus on love or any of its specific qualities. To do this, simply engage in conscious breathing and focus on one of the heart-based qualities of Agape, found in Chapter 19.

By raising your vibration, you will become sensitive to energy. It will be easier to recognize when upsets or disturbances seep into your energetic space. If you suddenly find yourself feeling disturbed or upset without provocation, you can return your focus and attention to conscious breathing and extricate yourself from the energy.

It is important to take action to disengage from thought form energy transference; otherwise you become a conduit, transferring the anger or disturbance to others. Gossip is a very common way to receive and transmit unhealthy thought form energy.

By actively focusing on thought forms that carry a higher frequency such as forgiveness, compassion, kindness, acceptance, trust, you insulate yourself from the unhealthy effects of lower-vibration thought forms such as anger, lust, greed, control or fear. Being engaged in loving thought forms enables you to maintain a high frequency when you come into contact with the lower frequencies of fearful thought forms and emotions.

Detaching from Fear-Based Thought Forms

Conscious breathing enables you to detach from fear-based thought forms and remain in your center. You will be unaffected by the upsets or disturbances of others.

Conscious breathing enables you to limit the length of your upsets. The longer you remain upset, the more difficult it becomes to regain your peace and serenity. Being upset also contributes to energetic disturbances lingering in the ethers. The sooner your focus and attention returns to conscious breathing, the sooner the seeds of unhealthy thought forms and their energy can be dissolved.

When you are focused on the breath, the peace and equanimity emanating from you will magnetically draw others to you who are at peace. It can also help dissolve the energy of disturbed thoughts and emotions spewing from those in your immediate proximity, provided they are willing to be affected.

By consistently focusing your thoughts on the heart-based qualities of love, others, especially those who are seeking peace, will find that their own agitation diminishes. If they are not open to feeling calm and centered, then your serenity will often magnetically repel them. If it does not, you are apt to walk away before you are affected.

EXERCISE:
HOW TO DETACH
FROM DIS-EASED THOUGHT FORMS

1. When dis-eased thoughts arise do not speak them; instead remain silent.

2. Return to conscious breathing.

3. Excuse yourself to a quiet private place. If none other is available, then use a bathroom for privacy and so that you do not disturb others.

4. Continue the centering process by praying with passion to shift the thought form energy from dis-ease to love.

5. Visualize pink to transmit unconditional love, green for healing and blue for peace. Saturate everyone involved in the disturbance with these colors, including you. For more information on colors, see the Appendix.

The Power of Maintaining Positive Thought Forms

Whenever disturbing thoughts arise, do not suppress or deny them. Doing so will lock the energy of the thoughts into some part of the physical body. Instead, engage in conscious breathing and practice detaching from the thought until you feel the disturbance subside. In addition, every time you replace a negative or unpleasant thought or emotion with a positive thought or emotion, the easier it becomes to do the next time. The more often you practice, the greater the likelihood that you will develop a habit of shifting disturbing thoughts and not allowing their energy to affect you.

Healing on all levels can and does occur by maintaining a state of positive focus in your thoughts and about your life. A study of "spontaneous" cancer remission undertaken by Dr. O. Carl Simonton, radiation oncologist in Fort Worth, Texas, revealed that all such patients had consistently held a positive idea (thought) that healing was taking place or had taken place. This particular thought form remained consistent regardless of what the patients considered the cause of healing.[1]

Affirmations, Bhajans and Mantras

Unhealthy habits grow out of the roots of unhealthy thoughts. A clear intention and a commitment to put that intention into action is required to free yourself from an unhealthy habit.

Affirmations, Bhajans and mantras are clear-intentioned, proactive statements, songs and chants. The power contained in an affirmation, Bhajan or mantra can be compared to an exponentially magnified prayer. When put into action with full focus, discipline and commitment to the Divine, their ability to influence and manifest desired changes is tremendous.

The Sacred Trinity of Passion, Will and Action Can Bring Affirmations to Fruition

Affirmations, Bhajans or mantras yield better results when you apply The Sacred Trinity of Radiant Health recipe of *Passion, Will and Action*. Take one component from each of the three bodies and mix them together to bring forth the fire of devotion and sincerity that provides opportunity for the affirmation to be realized.

The emotional body's healthy fire of Passion sparks your imagination, enabling you to create a powerful affirmation of change. The mental body's Will steels the mind, enabling you to focus on the affirmation and discipline yourself to use it. The physical body's component, action, keeps you moving proactively toward the goal of creating change. Consistent action increases the chance that the affirmation will produce the desired result. Used together, Passion, Will and Action create a solid foundation for change.

Uncovering the Resistance to Change

For an affirmation to be effective, you must first ascertain what the unhealthy habit provides. Often, the habit provides a sense of comfort, security or familiarity. Unhealthy habits always provide a benefit, otherwise they would be abandoned. If the benefits are not uncovered, change is unlikely, regardless of how often the affirmation is repeated. When the habit's underlying benefits are not identified, acknowledged and released, the affirmation will yield no results. The lack of change results from the ego's ability to justify the habit because of its superficial benefits, and erect a wall of resistance that renders your Passion and Will impotent, negating your desire to take action.

A common belief is that emotions stem from thoughts; and so by simply changing your thoughts, an unhealthy habit can be broken.

This does not work.

To create lasting change, the belief systems and emotions that impede your ability to effectively facilitate change need to be identified. Once identified, the mental body element, Will, which is a catalyst for change, can be used to sow the seeds of a healthy new thought pattern. This is one step in the process to break an unhealthy habit. Additionally, affirmations and a shift in posture, powered by Will, can help to discharge the electro-magnetic energy of emotions that get stored in the physical body.

Affirmations and Integration

Using a physical body movement with Passion to express a pro-active affirmation has integrative properties. The action creates a shift in the physical body's biochemistry releasing more endorphins and peptides. This, in turn, stimulates the emotional creative energy, enhances mental focus and clarity and produces more physical energy. This action integrates the three bodies.

By declaring your affirmation proactively and with Passion, as if you already have it, the first step to manifest change is set in motion. This occurs even though the affirmation might not be true at the moment it is being written and spoken. The next step is to apply your Will and take Action.

As you know, past experiences are a major contributor to belief systems, especially what you learned from your parents and what you witnessed. For example, if your parents struggled with money or taught you that money is the root of all evil, then it does not matter how many positive affirmations are written or spoken—such as *"money flows to me," "money is my friend"* or *"I have plenty of money"*—your money issues will not abate until your beliefs are addressed and changed. Only then will the seeds of the new affirmation have power to take root. If money or anything else is an emotional issue for you, try this exercise:

1. Write down everything you remember being taught overtly or covertly about the issue. Include what you learned from home, religion, friends, neighbors and teachers.

2. Write down your earliest recollections of how you felt about the issue. How did your learning about the issue affect your current belief systems?

3. After you have identified the belief systems and emotions, write down the good things that have come from the issue.

4. Write proactive affirmations about the issue that address the emotional charge you have with it. Put them into practice with the help of Passion, Will and Action.

When the thought forms that arise from belief systems and emotions are identified, owned and expressed, the affirmations will be more likely to clearly demonstrate a change in your self-awareness. The change will translate into the adopting of healthy new belief systems and the emotional charge associated with the issue will be dissolved.

Bhajans

A Bhajan is a sacred song of devotion. Bhajans are sung directly to a specific deity, master or to God Itself. Bhajans are sung by religious and Spiritual people all over the world. Bhajans are God-praising or God-invoking songs that are used as a tool to keep the mind's focus and attention on the Divine. All that you need to perform a Bhajan is a heart-felt desire to sing to God and a good song. Sing the song to God with all the Passion you can muster and its heart-felt vibrations reach through the ethers directly to the Divine.

Mantras

A mantra is a sacred syllable, word or phrase, chanted repeatedly in silence or aloud, in devotion to God. The intention of chanting a mantra is to focus the mind on the Divine. Chanting properly raises your vibration, and leads to self-realization. Affirmations can be turned into mantras by focusing on an issue, invoking the name of God or a realized master and chanting for the highest good. For example, one might chant, *"Jesus show me how to love,"* or *"God align my will with Your will"* or *"Allah provides me with everything."* The surrender of your personal desires, as well as dedicating your efforts to Spirit, does not mean you give up your dreams. It simply means that you release your attachment to a specific outcome as a result of your effort.

Mantras give the mind a specific task on which to focus. Mantras help eliminate subconscious mental chatter and wandering thoughts. With the mind steadfastly engaged in a mantra, attachments, agitations, anxieties and upsets melt away. Mantras can be used to raise your vibration and surround you with a shield that repulses fear-based thought forms. Traditionally, people of many faiths and religions have used mantras as a method to enter into Divine ecstatic communion with Spirit.

EXERCISE:
HOW TO TURN AN AFFIRMATION
INTO A MANTRA

1. Choose a habit you want to cultivate.

2. Write out a few positive affirmations about the habit.

3. Memorize one of the affirmations and use it in conjunction with a Passion-based physical movement.

4. Repeat the affirmation with Passion consistently during the day to support the new habit.

5. Turn the affirmation into a mantra by asking Spirit to support the new habit. Use the mantra in conjunction with meditation. The best time to meditate is 4 to 6 AM when the world and mind are calm and quiet.

6. Do not entertain any negative fear-based thoughts. When they arise, immediately return to the mantra. Chant the mantra with Passion until the mind is saturated and you feel calm and centered.

A Final Note on Affirmations and Mantras

It takes time for an affirmation or mantra to turn an unhealthy habit into a healthy habit and these three keys can help. One, use Passion in conjunction with the mantra. Two, use it consistently, and three, take Action.

Unhealthy habits are not broken in one day, nor are healthy habits formed in one day. Keep working at it until you experience the shift.

Do not give up if change is not immediate.

For example, if you are habitually late, use the affirmation, *"I am always on time."* Write a few affirmative statements about being on time and always emphasize the positive. For example, state, *"I am always on time"* rather than *"I am never late."* The Action of writing will also help to imprint a new memory pattern in the cellular structure.

Commit the written affirmation to memory, and use it frequently and with Passion. Also use your Will to take Action. For example, set the alarm and get up when it goes off, buy a watch, and leave early enough to be on time.

As you apply the affirmations and mantras, they will magnetize positive vibrations, unhealthy habits will be broken and healthy habits will be established.

22

Information

The next fundamental component in the outer layer of the mental body is information. TV, newspaper, radio or the internet are generally thought to be the primary sources of information. However, the root source of information is the senses. From the senses come all first-hand experiences and, like everything else in nature, the senses follow the principle of Yin and Yang. The five Yang senses—sight, sound, smell, taste and touch—identify the external/active information sources; while the five Yin senses—intuition, instinct, feelings, dreams and psychic ability such as extra sensory perception (ESP)—identify the internal/receptive information sources.

Information can be defined as a series of electro-magnetic waves that are transmitted through the ethers. When the waves of vibration reach another electro-magnetic body of energy, they are felt and then interpreted. Because these waves resonate at a specific rate of vibration, their energy can affect your body's frequency. In this way, information can have a direct and profound impact on your health and well-being.

Heart-based information emits a high frequency.

Ego-based information emits a low frequency.

The higher the frequency, the greater the possibility for health and well-being. The lower the frequency, the greater the possibility for pain, suffering and dis-ease.

The Effects of Outside Information

The need to be cognizant of your sources of information cannot be stressed enough. Information that enters through your external senses, whether you pay attention to it or not—like falling asleep while listening to the radio or TV—is absorbed into your subconscious and can influence your thoughts, emotions and behaviors. The way information affects your thoughts, feelings and actions can be blatant and subtle, either raising or lowering your vibration. Therefore, it is wise to be discriminating in the quantity and quality of your information sources. This is the reason that sages encourage you to read, speak, think, listen to and meditate on material with a Spiritual content.

To support Radiant Health, your information sources should stimulate physical, mental, emotional and Spiritual growth. They should promote balance and harmony, and provide you with an opportunity to learn more about yourself and others.

Unfortunately, the most easily accessible sources of information, such as mainstream commercial TV, radio, magazines and newspapers, normally do not elevate your Spiritual awareness, promote harmony and balance or improve health and well-being.

Take mainstream corporate-run commercial television news, for example. The excessive violence and tragedy portrayed by the mainstream commercial media as news does not uplift or inspire. It appeals to the lowest common denominator, the viewer's sense of curiosity and morbidity, which boosts ratings and advertising costs. This corporate ideology does nothing to promote health.

To the contrary, the emotional effects are experienced as deeper feelings of fear, insecurity and anxiety. Certainly there is a need to know about suffering so action can be taken to find and implement solutions. But rather than empowering feelings of hope, inspiration, strength and esteem, the mainstream media create feelings of powerlessness, hopelessness and depression by emphasizing and dramatizing suffering.

Balance can be achieved by reporting more inspirational and uplifting stories. But violence and sensationalism, not love and inspiration, sells advertising and boosts ratings. The way to create change is to stop consuming violence and sensationalism. When enough momentum is created the media, which reflects the collective consciousness, will stop presenting them.

Restoring personal and world balance requires a whole-hearted examination of information that perpetuates fear and hatred towards our environment, and our sisters and brothers. In the late '60s the rallying cry *"Make love not war"* was considered a radical and unattainable goal, but it is an idea and message whose time has come. Regardless of what the mainstream media report, the disparity between the rich and the poor, third world and industrialized nations, has reached epidemic proportions.

It is time to advocate the promotion of information that emphasizes holistic health and interdependence. It is time to applaud and support—with dollars, time and resources—individuals and businesses that use information to solve problems rather than dramatize them.

On a positive note, a growing number of alternative healing and consciousness-raising information sources are now finding a niche. Holistic health magazines and journals, personal growth and Spiritual literature, lectures, seminars and workshops, including Yoga studios, are springing up everywhere. By supporting them, you can make love, not war a reality.

The Effects of Inside Information

The Yin senses detect subtle energetic changes in frequency. When the Yang senses are overstimulated, the signals emitted by the Yin senses become difficult to identify. The Yin senses alert you to change and are a direct link to Spirit and higher realms of consciousness. Because the Yin senses correlate to the truth centers, they enable you to perceive the subtle energies of sentient non-physical beings such as Guides, Angels and Masters. This is a definition of "inside information."

Western science does not have the means to validate the Yin senses—standardized tests do not produce consistent results. However, everyone, including and especially children, has access to the Yin senses. Individuals who exhibit more developed forms of ESP are often viewed as odd. This perception is due in part to the fact that few of us have been taught anything about the Yin senses, much less how to develop them. Like any muscle, the Yin senses require stimulation to strengthen them; otherwise, they, too, will atrophy.

But things are changing.

Since the infamous UFO incident in Roswell, New Mexico in 1947, cases that involve Yin sense phenomena have been documented with increasing regularity. First-hand reports of UFO activity worldwide has steadily increased and more and more people report having had actual contact with extraterrestrials. People with impeccable credentials have written books that substantiate the existence of extraterrestrial beings, such as *Roswell, The Day After*, by Colonel Philip Corso—the man responsible for engineering the military cover-up of the UFO crash in Roswell, New Mexico. Others recount visions or visitations from ascended Masters such as Jesus of Nazareth, Mother Mary, Buddha, Krisna, Lao Tze or other Spiritual masters. Still others report that they have had clairvoyant, clairaudient and clairsentient experiences.

The increase in sensitivity to the Yin senses heralds an increase in conscious awareness.

The Yin Senses, Higher Vibration and Information

This increase in Yin sense activation has correlated with the increase in planetary vibration rate that resulted from the Harmonic Convergence on August 16, 1987 (see "Mayan Prophecy" in Chapter 2). As the vibratory rate continues to increase, more information can be received and contained. The process is similar to what happens when the vibration of a molecule speeds up. The faster it moves, the more it expands and the greater area it encompasses.

As the result of a quickening in the vibration rate, more people than ever are accessing and comprehending higher conscious information. In part this explains the increase in witnessing and reporting of extraordinary cosmic events. Conscious breathing can also stimulate the development of the Yin senses.

Complement the Yang Senses with the Yin Senses

The outwardly directed Yang senses—TV, radio, internet, etc.—on the other hand, shift your focus and attention away from your Spiritual center, placing it on the sensual, temporal pleasures of the external world. There is nothing inherently wrong with experiencing external beauty and pleasure. However, without active Yin senses, no balance can exist. Without balance, you run the risk of becoming enslaved to external desires. The end products are addictions, obsessions, compulsions and attachments.

Unlike the Yang senses, which alert you to the dense external energies of physical reality, the internal Yin senses are not as tangible. Because the Yin senses detect subtle energy rather than dense physical energy, it takes time to trust that what is being perceived is also real.

The outer layer mental body component, information, is the complementary counterpart to the outer layer emotional body component, experiences. The majority of your belief systems stem from your experiences, with others rooted in what we have been taught. Unhealthy environments imprint unhealthy belief systems that are expressed in unhealthy patterns of behavior and habits. These behaviors and habit patterns destroy relationships, diminish self-esteem and stop you from manifesting your dreams.

Consciousness-raising information can help you identify the limiting or fear-based belief systems that cause suffering. Gathering new information and putting it into action starts the process that leads to the disintegration of unhealthy imprinted belief systems and habits.

Often, when new to the Spiritual path, people will turn to mind-altering substances to activate the Yin senses. The exercise on the following page will help you to get in touch with the Yin senses naturally. Activate the Yin senses and you will raise your awareness and balance the Yang senses.

EXERCISE:
GATHERING INFORMATION
FROM NON-ORDINARY SOURCES

1. Disengage from all traditional forms of information such as TV, radio, newspaper, internet, talking or reading for one day.

2. Get out to a quiet spot in nature.

3. Detach from your thoughts and emotions.

4. Pick a tree, rock, mountain, stream, fish, bird or other animal and silently or aloud ask that source if you can commune, or be at one, with it.

5. Practice being with nature. Using the Yin senses, listen to nature and observe it in detail.

When you finish, write your experiences in a journal. Answer the following questions:

• What kind of information, such as history, stories or direct advice, did you receive?

• Was there a particular piece of information that affected how you perceive the world?

• How did it feel to go without your usual sources of information?

• Did you experience peace?

23

The Power of Will

Habits are formed over time and by constant repetition. When a thought form arises and is continually fed energy, the thought form solidifies and a habit is formed. It can take the average person up to eight years to establish a habit[1], but the process can be accelerated when the power of Will is put to use. The power of Will generates an unparalleled quantity of focused energy that you can use to manifest change in your life.

Will is the mental body's complementary partner of the emotional body component, Passion. Each is capable of producing a tremendous amount of energy. Will also is the most Yang element in the mental body and when the power of Will is well directed, your focus becomes laser sharp.

The power of Will propels you towards your goals, enabling you to persevere with determination against overwhelming odds and beyond all obstacles to accomplish seemingly impossible tasks. For example, a fire walk ceremony requires an individual to walk across searing, red-hot coals. Before walking across the coals, the Will is invoked to completely narrow the mind's focus in order to transcend the extreme heat of the coals and walk across the coals without being burned.

The Power of Will Charges the Body with Vital Energy

When invoked, the power of Will draws its vital energy from the electroprotonic center of the body's cells and from reservoirs of food energy that are stored in the brain.[2] If more energy is needed, the cosmic source brings it directly to the body through the medulla[3], instantly charging every atom with the power of life force energy.

Additional energy can be obtained from the cosmic source by maintaining a willing and joyful attitude. When you willingly engage in action, happily performing a given task, you will feel far more energized. When the task is complete, you might be in need of rest, but you will not experience the exhaustion that results from resistance.

The power of Will can be tempered by a commitment to use it to carry out the highest good. This includes using it to eradicate unhealthy habits, perform loving actions and propel you to self-realization.

Will Can Also Deplete the Body's Vital Energy

When invoked by fear, Will activates the adrenal glands, flooding the body with adrenaline, supplying the energy needed to complete the immediate task. But when the task is completed, the body is left depleted. When fueled by fear, other ego-based emotions such as greed, impatience, anger and lust rise to the surface and the faculties of reason and right action are either seriously impaired or become totally inoperative.

Invoking fear-based Will can enable you to attain a goal, but seldom does its use end with positive results. The exception to the rule occurs when a parent, overcome by fear, is able to lift an otherwise unmovable object off of his/her stricken child. Otherwise, fear-based Will overwhelmingly results in more pain and suffering.

When questions arise about the proper use of Will, for example, *"Am I engaged in self-centered Will or Divine Will?"*, prayer and meditation can help you uncover the answer. When guided by love, the Divine Will will always be carried out.

When you feel unclear about your direction or actions, use the exercise below to align with the Divine Will and express your highest truth and put love into action.

EXERCISE:
ALIGNING WITH THE DIVINE WILL

1. Write down your desired outcome as it pertains to a specific situation such as changing jobs or moving.

2. Be willing to surrender your desired outcome.

3. Affirm that your desire is to align with the highest Will.

4. Pray for knowledge of the Divine Will and the ability to carry it out.

5. Meditate, opening your heart to receive the Divine Will. When you receive the answer it will resonate with love.

6. Put the answer you receive into action.

When invoked, the Divine Will will always present you with love-based guidance and actions. If the guidance or actions you receive are not based in love then self-Will is at work. Being honest and acting with integrity is key to the process of aligning with the highest Will. When your heart is open, you can identify and then release any self-centered desires. When you are free of doubt, confusion or fear, your actions will be love-based, and your personal Will will be in alignment with the Divine Will.

In this state you will feel the love of the Divine flowing through your being and you can be confident that your actions will harm no one, including yourself. You will also know that your actions will be of great benefit to all those to whom they are directed.

-24-

The Ego

Every human being is comprised of two dynamic, expressive components. The two are Spirit, which resides in the heart and expresses your divine nature, and ego, which resides in the mind and expresses your human personality. Spirit is congruent with the light, while ego is congruent with the dark. Learning to access and embody Spirit enables you to experience Radiant Health. The ego is the element that stands between you and the experience of Radiant Health.

Directing your focus and attention to the inner journey to Spirit enables you to open your heart and realize your true nature. Yet, the ego commands your attention when you do not follow Spirit's path, maintain an open heart, seek guidance before acting or work to increase your self-awareness. The ego will seize the opportunity to shift your focus to the external-material path of the temporal world. Although the material path can be fun and pleasurable, if you are not well grounded on an inner path of awareness, you will experience the ego ups and downs that are the root of suffering.

The ego has a complex and lavish armamentarium of defense mechanisms. These include the ego behaviors and the three ego components of separation, which you will learn about in Chapters 26 and 27. However, before its defenses can be overcome, it is important to realize that the ego, an inherent part of the human personality, can be expelled or exorcised. As the element that stands opposite of Spirit, it would appear that the ego preserves the balance found in duality. Duality, however, is total illusion, and the point is to transcend duality.

Spirit always stands strong, but often silent.

Until consciously called upon, Spirit will remain veiled behind the ego.

The greatest challenge on *The Journey to Radiant Health* is to learn to identify the ego in all of its disguises, and liberate yourself from its dis-ease-producing characteristics. The first step is recognizing egoistic attitudes, perceptions, thoughts, belief systems and other defense mechanisms. They comprise the roots of suffering.

The second is to employ your Will to change them. By engaging in the process to identify, unravel and detach from the ego personality, Spirit can be unveiled and accessed. Then you will realize that you are interwoven and interdependent with everyone and everything. When the ego personality is mastered, suffering will take a back seat to the peace, happiness, harmony and joy that are inherent in Spirit.

The Ego and Pain and Suffering

The ego is the root cause of suffering although it does not necessarily control the circumstances from which pain arises. Pain is a natural part of life, and is intrinsic to any path of growth. Pain is often experienced at the point when that which no longer serves you needs to be shed. Suffering is a direct result of the ego's resistance to letting go, and judgment of pain.

Ego reactions to pain are the ultimate cause of suffering.

At its core, suffering results from the ego's ability to create the appearance that you (can) exist separately from pain or others. This egoistic belief distorts reality, provoking reactions to anything that appears different or threatens the status quo. Judgments and resistance are characteristic ego behaviors. The greater the judgment of pain, the greater the resistance to pain. The greater the resistance to pain, the greater the suffering. Resistance to feeling pain is at the root of repression and denial. But pain is information. When you experience pain, it is informing you that something is happening. Most often, pain is a signal that something is out of balance.

Pain needs to be acknowledged and its roots uncovered.

But the avoidance, repression and denial of pain—whether it be physical, mental or emotional—has turned into an epidemic in American society. Get a headache, take an aspirin. Pop another pill when you experience heartburn, insomnia, drowsiness, stress or tension. Even the pain associated with childbirth is not immune to suppression. Caesarean sections have become routine money-making procedures. Epidurals and other anesthetizing drugs are administered to avoid pain without considering the long-range effects on the baby.

However, pain is still, at its root level, energy. As you learned earlier, energy—in this instance pain—cannot truly be avoided, repressed or denied. At some point in time, the repressed or denied pain will rise to the surface, manifesting as dis-ease.

Understanding the Ego

Learning how the ego operates is the first step towards ego mastery. A number of different perspectives will be used to examine the ego and gain a greater understanding of it, starting with the perspective of the ego as the shadow self.

The Ego As the Shadow Self

The dark side of human nature is selfish and impure, chaotic and without reason, unable to know or express love and truth. It is filled with every destructive element that can be imagined. The shadow side hides the thoughts and emotions that we do not want to admit having, while also being the element that attaches to and obsesses on those same thoughts and emotions. From the shadow emanates every form of fear that can be imagined, created or acted out.

A common temptation is to repress or deny the existence of the shadow self. Any attempt to vanquish it, however, will simply result in the compartmentalizing and fragmenting of the ego-personality. Disintegration at this core level leads to emotional, mental and/or physical dis-ease. The shadow can be abolished, but to do so, it is crucial to realize that you have authority over it. In the East, it is said that the mind is a wonderful servant, but a terrible master. This is because the mind is home to the ego. In the upcoming chapters, you will learn how to manage your shadow self and become the ego's master rather than its servant.

The Ego As a Mental Body Component

The ego's energy, viewed from the perspective of it being a component in the mental body, moves in a linear direction. The ego commonly directs its energy in an outward movement. The ego, being a mental body element, is limited to a perceived reality in which everything is composed of, and defined by, two points: a starting point and an ending point. The linear orientation of the mental body's energy prohibits the ego from being able to comprehend anything as being whole and complete, or without beginning or end, or perfect as it is. It also prohibits the ego from being able to see and comprehend a multitude of differing viewpoints.

The limitations of duality essentially confine the ego to very narrow parameters of perception. Because the ego operates in the restricted and illusory field of dualism and polarities, it defines everything as either itself, or not itself. This shortcoming causes the ego to perceive and describe everything in dualistic terms: right or wrong, black or white, important or insignificant, good or bad, or you or me.

This perception produces the valid, but untrue, feelings of separation that produce confusion, opposition and conflict—in you, or between you and others. In the ego's defense, however, it is only fulfilling its primary purpose.

The Ego's Primary Purpose

The ego, pure in its nature, has one simple agenda: to fulfill its primary purpose. *The ego's primary purpose is to ensure your survival.* As the ego's master, your responsibility is to understand that it only acts to carry out its duty. This means that you need to be aware of, and face, any arising fears that threaten your survival. When a fear threatens your emotional, mental or physical survival, the ego will carry out its purpose with zeal. It will defend you from any threat, regardless of whether the threat is real or imagined, or whether the attack comes from within or outside.

For example, if you realize that eating when you feel upset is unhealthy, you might decide to try to adopt a healthy pattern such as feeling and expressing the upset rather than eating to suppress it. The ego, being unfamiliar with the healthy new pattern of behavior, will perceive the change, as well as its challenges and ramifications, as a threat to the status quo, and therefore to your emotional survival. The ego will do everything in its power to sabotage your efforts.

Confined by the limitations of duality, anything the ego perceives as the unknown, or as not being part of itself, is defined as a threat and will be attacked unless you intervene.

The fear-based ego always externalizes its focus—projecting a threat as being something other than itself. In the previous example, the threat was a behavior, but it can be as simple as skin color, gender, class, attitude or style, or as complex as projecting things that do not exist. Complex fears include the belief that people are out to get you, that places are unsafe or other unfounded phobias.

The Ego Needs a Master

The ego, because it has the ability to attack and do harm to you and others, can be likened to an untrained dog. Although a dog should always receive love, attention and care, it also should be trained to obey its master's commands. Failure to assert yourself as the ego's master enables it to run amok. Then the ego recklessly reacts to your every fear, attacking everything that seemingly poses a threat to your survival.

It is important to understand that fear and ego are completely enmeshed. Where one exists, the other is sure to be found. Realizing that fear and the ego are inextricably bound is a powerful step in the process to master the ego.

Your ability to master the ego
is primarily dependent on developing the ability
to accept and embrace it.

Squarely face your fears, and regardless of whether you overcome them, their power will diminish and the ego will become compliant to your commands. Take this action and you will transcend the ego's dualistic world of polarities.

Fear

Whenever you experience fear, you have an opportunity to achieve a greater degree of personal growth and self-mastery. Fear is intrinsic to the ego. Paradoxically, because it is goal oriented and driven, the ego exacerbates the perception that if you do not overcome your fears, then you can only be viewed as a failure.

This is a typical linear ego viewpoint, and it is wholly untrue.

The growth you experience when you face your fears is not dependent on whether you overcome them. The fruit of your labor is in the effort put forth. Make the commitment to face your fears and in time (and with hard work) you will be victorious.

Left unchecked, fear can arrest your drive and motivation. Fear can imprison you in the comfort zone of familiarity that keeps you from taking risks and challenging yourself to expand and evolve beyond ego-imposed limitations.

Fear can also cause you to employ the ego behaviors, found in Chapter 26, as well as the components of separation—rationalization, justification and manipulation—found in Chapter 27. These fool you into believing that you are acting from love when in truth your actions are deeply rooted in fear.

Being a constrictive and contracting energy, fear thwarts your ability to define your higher purpose and stand in the power of love. Fear strangles initiative and promotes denial, resistance, procrastination and other debilitating emotional attitudes that promote dis-ease.

To recognize the impairing effects of fear and liberate yourself from them, fear must be identified, owned and expressed. Concealed fears will subconsciously control you, impeding or arresting your ability to overcome obstacles on the path to your dreams.

In the quest to identify and face your fears, the three bodies—

emotional, mental and physical—can provide helpful clues because each body displays specific symptoms whenever fear is present.

Physically: when fear is present, the breath is either held or becomes erratic, spastic or choppy; the stomach gets queasy and the body trembles or becomes tense; and the need to eliminate in either a bowel movement or urination is immediate.

Mentally: when fear is present, your conscious awareness and ability to be fully present in the moment diminishes considerably; confusion sets in and you will become intellectually stifled or over-talkative.

Emotionally: when fear is present, you will feel ungrounded, losing your center and confidence, as well as the ability to manage your emotions. You will feel nervous or anxious and become reactive towards others and suspicious of everyone and everything in your environment.

The Two Core Beliefs behind Fear

All ego actions are motivated by fear. Fear is a product of forgetting or being unable to recognize the Divine perfection and order that exist in every moment and interaction. To counteract the ego actions caused by fear, it is of vital importance to use the power of Will to restrain the ego and bring it under your command.

Fear can be traced to one of two core beliefs. The first belief is you are powerless to change. The second belief is something of value can or will be taken from you. Neither belief is true. Nonetheless, each can and will continue to affect your thoughts, emotions and ability to take action until it is faced, examined, and dismissed because it is not truth.

The First Core Belief: You Are Powerless to Change

Although you have no power to change others, and at times you have no power to change your external circumstances, you always have the power to change yourself.

You can choose to change in any moment, in any situation.

Fear is a real and valid emotion that can be overwhelming at times. To realize your potential, do not let fear stop you. When you are gripped by fear, you can change. This is why the first core belief is untrue.

To overcome fear, construct a course of loving actions. For example, as soon as you recognize fear being aroused in you, practice step one: *conscious breathing*. Gently reinforce the knowledge that you create your reality and be determined to identify, own and face your fears. You have the power to pour the expansive energy of love into every thought, emotion and action, and change your attitude and perceptions. The work can be quite confrontive and challenging, but it can be done. Do not reinforce any fear-based belief about being powerless such as *"I cannot do that."* Instead, empower yourself by using phases like *"Yes I can!"* or *"I will find a way."* State the affirmative phrases emphatically, with the energy of determination, commitment, Passion and Will.

Even when it is hard to believe, act as if you do.

The more energy you put into it, the more confidence you will build. As Spirit in human form, you are endowed with the power and ability to manifest magnificence and splendor.

With a little hard work, you can make anything happen!

The Second Core Belief:
Something You Value Can Be Taken from You

The truth is material possessions, freedom or even your life can be taken from you. The pursuit of your life's purpose might even cost you some or all of these things. Those who have authority over you—such as parents, bosses, police, teachers, judges and government officials—might deprive you of your valued possessions. But the freedom to choose how you will act can never be taken from you.

Whether you respond with love or react from fear is solely your choice. The body can be chained and shackled, but no one can shackle the mind or force you to think or feel the way they want.

Consider the courage of former South African president Nelson Mandela. Stripped of everything and imprisoned for 27 years, he stood tall and remained impeccable. Never did he relinquish or betray his ideals and beliefs, nor could anyone take them from him or force him to surrender them.

His love, vision and determination to see South Africa become an integrated and free nation were never compromised. He looked squarely in the face of a death sentence—death is one of the greatest fears the ego can manifest—and resolved to stand in the power of his heart's truth. He lived to realize his dream.

Other courageous visionaries also fought fearlessly for South Africa's freedom, including Steven Biko, but did not live to realize the dream. However, because they squarely faced the fear of death and accepted it as a distinct possibility when they chose to engage in the struggle, their lives were not taken from them.

Facing Your Fears

When faced with fear, do your best to exemplify courage and impeccability. Focus the power of your Will and intention on carrying forth the highest truth. Seek to break the chains of fear with every tool available to you, and your actions will inspire others to stand for their heart's truth. As in the immortal words spoken by Sir Winston Churchill, *"Never. Never. Never. Never. Never give in."* [1]

Even if you fall short of the mark, do not give in. Otherwise, the ego experiences an externalized form of death through the loss of identity, image and appearance. Fear often rears its head at a crossroads in life, when you are experiencing the stress of a major change. Whether you are successful or not, facing your fears demonstrates courage and provides rich opportunities for personal and Spiritual growth.

Dispelling fear is a process, so try not to get trapped by the ego's desire for instant results. Use common sense and do not bite off more than you can chew. If you try to do too much too fast, you might fall into the ego trap of false bravado or machismo—acting courageous and unafraid when in reality you are afraid. This is self-deceptive and can cause more suffering, figuratively or literally.

Any time you feel fear, it can be used as an opportunity for personal growth.

EXERCISE:
DISSOLVE YOUR FEAR—PART I

1. When you feel fear, identify and own it.

2. Return to conscious breathing. Take long, slow, deep inhales and exhales. Double the count on the exhale.

3. Recite a mantra with Passion and Will to dissolve the fear. Mantra suggestions are *"Spirit always takes care of me"* or *"God is in me and with me."*

4. When you feel mentally clear, physically energized and emotionally centered, take action. You might still feel some fear, but you can take action before it dissolves completely.

EXERCISE:
DISSOLVE YOUR FEAR—PART II

1. Determine which one of fear's two core beliefs you are experiencing:
   A. Fear that you are powerless to change.
   B. Fear that something of value can be taken from you.

2. Acknowledge that the ego is trying to ensure your survival.

3. Affirm that you have the power to change.

4. Use your Will to shift your attention from fear to love.

5. Pray and meditate to find loving solutions to expel fear.

It is counterproductive to try and force yourself to conquer your fear. Rather than taking actions when you are not ready, willing, able or prepared, try to strengthen your resolve to act in a loving and truthful manner. Try opening your heart and admit when you feel afraid, unsure or insecure. Being compassionate with yourself as you attempt to overcome your fears will dissipate some of the pressure that is a natural part of facing challenges.

In relationship to the ego fear that something can be taken from us, we alluded to two more ego fears: the fear of death and the loss of our identity, image or appearance. Let us explore each in greater detail.

Death

Life and death make up nature's greatest dualistic cycle. Everything that is born eventually will die. Death, which is often thought of as an ending, is the Yin element that balances the Yang element, life. As a Yin element, one's death is a Spiritual and sacred event marking the completion of the Yang cycle of life. It is a time to bear witness as your loved ones transition from this worldly dimension to the next. It is also a ceremonial time to honor the closure of one's life journey and departure from the physical plane.

A healthy and loving heart can acknowledge death as a natural transition. It is viewed as a shift from one state of consciousness to another. However, from the ego perspective, the Spiritual significance of transition is non-existent. Death instead is marked by pain and trauma, doubt and confusion. To the linear-natured ego, death signifies the end rather than a transition. Death becomes something to fear, deny and avoid at all costs.

To a large extent, this is why our culture sends our dying to institutions. We have learned to fear death. We also deny and disassociate ourselves from pain; and because death is associated with pain, we have trouble acknowledging death as being a natural and beautiful transition to life.

On a more esoteric level, the fear is associated with death because we have lost sight of the reality that our true essence is Spirit. This is easy to understand in light of dogmas that are used to create fears about what awaits us in the great beyond. It can be difficult enough to feel trust that our Spirit continues to exist after the physical body expires, without adding fear-based beliefs about what might happen to us once we get there. Still, physical death is not the only kind of death the ego fears.

To the Ego, Change Is Synonymous with Death

There are a wide variety of ego deaths that you can experience, and while all are illusory they are all valid. For example, you can die of fright, shame, guilt and embarrassment. But change represents stepping into the unknown, and because the greatest fears arise from projections of the unknown, the ego associates change with death.

The ego experiences change as a threat to that which is comfortable and familiar, essentially a threat to your survival. It is important to recognize that familiarity and comfort are key to the ego's survival. Otherwise, when you want to replace unhealthy habits with healthy ones, the ego will sabotage your attempts to change. The ego will continually utilize its components of separation and ego characteristics in an effort to maintain the status quo, regardless of whether the familiar and comfortable patterns have outgrown their usefulness and are causing you to suffer or are limiting your growth,

The ego can cause you to cling to unhealthy relationships, behaviors and habits because change represents death. When you are ready to make healthy changes in your life, honor the death of that which you are releasing and acknowledge the fears associated with the changes, and you will master the ego.

Counteracting the Ego's Fear of Death

Declare the three truths below and you can mitigate the paralyzing effects caused by the ego's fear of death.

1. *I have everything I need right here in this moment.*

In every moment and in every situation you have everything you need. Needs sustain life: food, water, air, warmth and shelter. Often, needs are confused with desires. Desires are the ego cravings that lead to suffering, especially when they are not being met.

2. *I am an infinite being, capable of creating all things.*

Although your Spirit dwells within a finite body, you are a manifestation of the Divine. As such, you are unlimited. You are fully capable of using your emotional body's energy to create, your mental body's energy to develop a plan of action and your Passion and Will to bring the plan to fruition.

What you believe in, is where your creative energy and power to manifest is directed. When you choose limiting beliefs you will manifest fear, obstacles, resistance and patterns of scarcity. When you choose limitlessness your creative energy will enable you to overcome obstacles and manifest your dreams.

3. *Death is an illusion.*

Although the pain and grief you feel for the loss of a loved one is valid, and should not be denied or repressed, there is no death— only transition and change. In every moment of your life, change takes place even though your Spirit/soul exists in an infinite state of timelessness.

In the Bhagavad Gita, the master Krisna says, *"The soul cannot be stamped out, burned, drowned or withered."*[2] Focus on your Spirit while you meditate and you will realize that you incarnated to have a broad range of human experiences. Meditate further and it will become clear to you that the ego fear of death is the only thing that can stop you from fully living.

Identity, Image and Appearance

On the stage of life, you experience a variety of identities: child, teen, adult, brother, sister, father, mother, friend, spouse, lover, teacher and student. The career you choose, whether it be doctor, lawyer or healer, also is a role you play. The roles are not who you are, they are simply part of the identity that you assume in your human experience.

The ego, perceiving you to be your identity, becomes attached to it. The ego places a tremendous amount of significance and importance on your identity. It can use your class, education, financial status, race, religion, looks and personality to create your identity.

It is easy to become invested in your identity. But when you become attached to your identity, the ego is in control. When things change—such as getting older or losing the things you identify as important—you will experience an identity crisis. Without a Spiritual foundation, the sense of security that enables you to adapt to changes and flow through them with ease will be lost. Without a solid foundation based in the knowledge of your true nature, who you are in the world becomes more important than who you are in reality.

The Toxic Effects of Youth Worship

One of the more widespread behaviors associated with the fear of death is becoming strongly identified with image and appearance. This has led to a cultural obsession with youth. Humanity has drifted so far from its roots in Spirit that growing old has become a dreaded fear. Old age is viewed as *"the end,"* and perceived as a disease to be avoided at all costs.

Traditionally, the elders of a culture were revered as bearers of wisdom and knowledge. But times have changed. Our elders are no longer admired as powerful and wise beings; they are viewed as weak and vulnerable. As a result, our elders are routinely institutionalized, and the youths that could most benefit from their wisdom have little opportunity to connect with them.

A more painful truth about the cultural desire to follow youth is that it clearly exposes the deficiency and scarcity of Spiritual wisdom and leadership displayed by post-modern elders. The renunciation of our elders, the glorification of youth and the overemphasis on image and appearance signify an underlying fear of death. This fear also manifests in elders that conform to youth worship to gain approval or feel accepted, comfortable or safe. When conformance takes precedence over being authentic and spontaneous, standing on principles or being willing to die for what you believe, it also signals an underlying fear of death. All in all, this leads to the decay of integrity, dignity, honor and wisdom.

Youth worship weakens society.

A dominant ego chooses image and appearance over honesty and humility. Mistakes, shortcomings and anything else that might tarnish the image, or create an appearance of vulnerability or weakness, will be ignored or denied.

When image and appearance become this important, the world of sensual pleasures, temptations and seductive appeal has distracted you from realizing your Spiritual nature. While you might find excitement and stimulation, lasting joy and fulfillment cannot be found in the world of sensual pleasures.

Emphasize the Similarities, Not the Differences

Practice seeing yourself in others and others in you and you can detach from ego identity, image and appearance—all of which underscore the fear of being the true Spirit that you really are. Emphasize similarities rather than differences. For example, everyone bleeds red blood, breathes air, feels emotions and wants to be happy. Differences in religion, skin color, class, race, gender, age, culture, nationality, social status or any other classification are superficial and do not make one better than another.

Follow these suggested actions and the ego is likely to cause upheaval in your life. Because the ego's primary purpose is to ensure your survival, it will view these actions as a threat to your sense of identity. The ego is incapable of understanding how it will survive if the identity is lost. However, find the similarities and you transcend the feeling of superiority, and weaken the ego's ability to keep you bonded to the lower nature personality.

We all sprout from the same seed, have the same human traits and characteristics, make the same mistakes and sometimes act from ego. Reduce the importance of image and appearance and it will be easier to serve others with compassion and humility. Take action, face your fears and stand in the light of your true identity, Spirit in human form.

Without action, nothing changes.

Never yield to fear, even if it is not immediately overcome, because each time a fear is identified, owned and expressed it loses a measure of its power.

Ego Behaviors

The ego behaviors listed below conceal fears such as insecurity, inadequacy or anxiety. As defense mechanisms, the ego behaviors hide from, repress, or protect us from identifying, owning and expressing the unhealthy range of emotions associated with sadness and anger.

The ego behaviors' primary purposes are to attack others, reinforce or exaggerate your own feelings of superiority, or sabotage your own self-esteem and self-worth.

EGO BEHAVIORS

judgment	envy	lust
blaming	pride	greed
opinions	vanity	worry
resistance	desires	deceit
ignorance	laziness	boredom
arrogance	impatience	negativity
resentment	martyrdom	selfishness
stubbornness	competition	attachments
self-deprecation	self-centeredness	expectations
	self-destruction	

The Seven Fear-Disguising Ego Behaviors

The seven fear-disguising ego behaviors are distinguished by characteristics that put them in a special classification. The main distinguishing characteristic is that these ego behaviors become established in the ego personality at a very young age. After they become fixed in the personality, the challenge is to eliminate them. Most often, this is a lifelong challenge.

While anyone at any time can act out any of the seven fear-disguising ego behaviors, two of the seven are prominent in the ego personality. Every individual is subject to two of the seven fear-disguising ego behaviors.

Carefully consider each of the seven, along with its corresponding fear. Be introspective and honest and you will uncover the primary and secondary fear-disguising ego behaviors that have been embedded in your personality. After you discover the fear-disguising ego behaviors, you can work to master them.

If you have trouble identifying the two, enlist the help of some trusted friends. Friends are often objective and can help you see beyond your own limitations.

Arrogance: disguises the fear of being vulnerable.

Impatience: disguises the fear of missing something.

Stubbornness: disguises the fear of change.

Greed: disguises the fear of not having enough.

Martyrdom: disguises the fear of being worthless.

Self-deprecation: disguises the fear of being inadequate.

Self-destruction: disguises the fear of loss of control.

How to Disengage from Ego Behaviors

All ego behaviors stem from fear and destroy truth. Fear resonates at a lower frequency, weakens the immune system, the central nervous system and the internal organs, and leaves you susceptible to dis-ease. When an ego behavior arises, it is a signal to stop what you are doing, return to conscious breathing and identify the fear that is triggering it.

As you become grounded in conscious breathing, the fear will become easier to identify. Identify and express the fear and you eliminate the need to engage in the ego behavior. Your heart will open and the feelings of peace, love and joy will return.

The Ego's Components of Separation

The ego also uses the reasoning intellect to hide fear and deny truth. In the intellect, the ego employs the three components of separation, *rationalization, justification and manipulation,* to distort truth, defend unscrupulous or selfish actions, attack the credibility of others or shift responsibility away from us and blame others for our predicaments.

One simple example is blaming traffic as the reason for being late to an appointment. Blaming is a rationalizing behavior.

To stop the ego from utilizing the components of separation, take responsibility for your actions, amend your errors and accept consequences when appropriate. For example, if you are going to be late for an appointment, admit to yourself that you did not leave early enough and call to say you are going to be late. Then admit your error to others and accept the consequences.

The following is a classic rationalizing thought: *"If only he/she would change, my problems would be solved and I would be happy."* This ego rationalization causes you to be a victim, which excuses you from taking responsibility or action to change your circumstances.

Defending your actions or inaction or blaming others are common justifying behaviors. Classic justifications of non-loving actions are: *"I hit him because he hit me first"* or *"If you are nice to me, I will be nice to you."* Justifying your actions stops you from changing your circumstances and behaviors. It also prohibits you from putting the highest truth, love, into action. When the urge arises to blame others, shift the focus back to yourself, identify what you need to change and put love into action.

The Three Components of Separation on a Larger Scale

Although we are moving towards the light, the effects of the ego (darkness) can be seen at work on a larger scale. In governments and corporations, individuals have the power to make decisions that affect the health and well-being of millions, perhaps billions, of people. When those in positions of corporate and government leadership wield the destructive power of even one of the ego's components of separation, the population at large suffers the consequences.

In today's society, it is difficult for political and corporate leaders to avoid the corrupting influence of the ego. The three components are regularly used to divert attention away from selfish and destructive agendas, minimize responsibility and accountability and ensure political and corporate survival.

Rationalization and Justification in the Corporate and Political Arenas

Consider the Environmental Protection Agency (EPA). The EPA sets and enforces public health and environmental standards. In the last 15 years, almost half of the EPA's top-level officials in the pesticides and toxics division left to work for corporate chemical companies or their lobbying firms.

These are the same companies the EPA is charged to regulate.

Between March 1993 and March 1995 a large number of trips for EPA employees were financed by mega–chemical corporate giants such as Ciba-Geigy, Monsanto, DuPont, Dow and organizations connected to these corporations.[1] The revolving door policy between EPA employees and the corporate chemical industry points to a conflict of interest. How can the EPA effectively regulate the chemical industry when the chemical industry is allowed to sponsor trips that could influence the decision-making process of EPA employees?

When concerns are voiced that the EPA's impartiality and integrity are being compromised, corporate and government officials defend themselves by *justifying* the practices. The public's concerns are dismissed by *rationalizing* these actions as if there is nothing to be concerned about in regards to these practices.

This is one example of the corporate and political ego epidemic.

Corporate and Political Manipulation

Many political and corporate leaders use the ego component of manipulation to acquire power, the political goal, or to maximize profits, the corporate goal. Manipulative tactics are used to gain the public's trust. For example, organizations with names like *The American Council on Science and Health, The Keep America Beautiful Campaign, The Information Council on the Environment, Consumer Alert* and *The National Wetlands Coalition* lead the public to believe that they were founded to protect and serve citizens and consumers.

In truth, corporations created and are funding these organizations.

These "front groups" were not established to protect the environment or the public's health; they were created to carry out the corporate agenda. Their objective is achieved by manipulating the public into believing that they serve the public interest.

As a case in point, consider the front group *The American Council on Science and Health.* The carefully chosen pro-consumer name belies the fact that it is being funded by corporate giants that include Monsanto, Burger King, Coca-Cola, PepsiCo, Nutrasweet, Nestle USA, Exxon, Union Carbide and Dow. The name lulls the public into a false sense of security, believing that its information is trustworthy, unbiased and serves the public's best interest. However, the executive director defends the nutritional value of fast foods, pesticides and dairy cow growth hormones.

Another front group, *The National Wetlands Coalition,* is a conglomeration of oil and gas companies, including Exxon, Shell and Mobil. This front group was created to battle and overcome legal challenges or any other obstacles that threaten its corporate members' rights to drill for oil in wetlands.

Most large corporations contribute to a multitude of these organizations. For example, in 1991 Dow Corporation was contributing to ten such front groups. The aforementioned front groups are just a few of the many organizations created by public relation firms and funded by corporations. Merrill Rose, executive vice-president of Porter/Novelli, a public relations firm, tells companies, *"Put your words in someone else's mouth."*[2]

Front groups do just that.

They employ lawyers, so-called scientists and other experts to publish reports and present information that back and publicly promote the corporate agenda. They create smoke screens by refuting research, documentaries and exposés that link corporations to deceptive and harmful actions. They also cause widespread confusion by attacking the character and integrity of those who expose self-serving corporate agendas. Ironically, they do all of this while claiming to represent the public interest.

This epitomizes the ego component of *manipulation* at work on a larger scale.

Power, and the Challenge to Master the Ego

Being in a position of power is arguably the greatest challenge on *The Journey to Radiant Health*. Power is seductive and presents plenty of temptations to engage in self-serving actions. To master the ego when you are in a leadership position, awareness is paramount. Act responsibly, be accountable and do not engage in ego behaviors or use the ego components of separation. These actions can be difficult, but you can meet the challenges of leadership. Stand in integrity and commit to serve others and promote the health and well-being of the planet.

A leader's struggle to engage in Dharma, *right action*, reflects the struggle that takes place in the hearts and minds of individuals from every walk of life. In the Koran, the prophet Mohammed describes the small and the great Jihads. The small Jihad is a battle that is fought when an enemy attacks your family. But, the great Jihad is the inner struggle to destroy the ego. The great Jihad has to be invoked by conscious intention, and is the most wholesome battle that can be waged.

Invoke the great Jihad.

Ask the Creator to guide your actions, help you face and overcome your fears and remove every ego obstacle (such as attitudes, perceptions, beliefs or experiences) that keep you from putting love into action.

If your hard work does not produce immediate results, do not give up.

Given the ego's predisposition to demand and expect instant gratification, it can provoke the negative polarity of skepticism—suspicion—when things do not go as you wish. If immediate results are not forthcoming, counteract the suspicion by utilizing the positive polarity of skepticism—investigation. Explore every possible avenue. Take risks and be flexible, open minded, patient, persistent and willing to change.

A Final Note on the Ego

Strive to be your best, but do not take yourself too seriously. Laugh more, and place less importance on your identity, image and appearance. Step closer to the truth of your Divine nature by letting go of attachments to your thoughts, beliefs, emotions and experiences. Do not allow the ego to make you to feel superior when you do well, or inferior when you fall short.

Take the middle road and forgo the ego's dramatic ups and downs.

The ego behaviors, the components of separation, the two core fears and their subset fears give you an index of the traits intrinsic to the ego personality. Use the detachment exercise on the following page to help you on the quest to master the ego and experience Radiant Health. Finally, consider these points relative to the ego:

- *When the ego arises, it is a signal that your need for love and attention has either gone unnoticed or is being ignored or denied.*

- *The ego is the only element that stops you from conveying love and truth in every action.*

- *View the ego neutrally, neither as friend nor enemy, and its power will fade.*

EXERCISE:
PRACTICING DETACHMENT

1. Identify and then write out a list of your attachments including relationships, thoughts, beliefs, material possessions, emotions, resentments, experiences and desires.

2. Pray for the ability to detach from your attachments and desires.

3. Do not entertain attachment- or desire-based thoughts and emotions. Whenever attachments or desires cause you to feel pain or to suffer, use your Will to shift your thoughts and emotions from attachments and desires to detachment and service.

4. Affirm that you have everything you need and that the universe is in perfect order.

fewer attachments = less pain and suffering

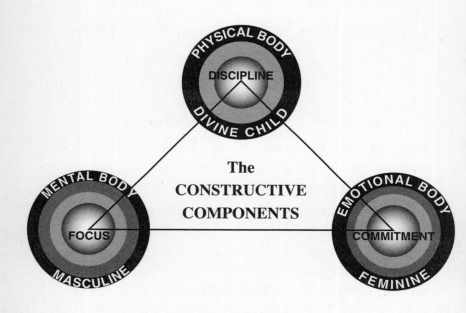

28

The Constructive Mental Body Components: Focus, Commitment, and Discipline

The constructive components provide the light of the masculine energy which is necessary to sustain a heightened level of conscious awareness. The constructive components keep you in alignment and communion with Spirit.

When used as an integrated and cohesive unit, each component expresses one of the specific characteristics of The Sacred Trinity of Radiant Health. Focus expresses masculine energy that provides clear direction and drive. Commitment expresses feminine energy that establishes and nurtures relationships. Discipline expresses the genderless Divine Child energy that devotes itself to a specific teaching or course of action. On *The Journey to Radiant Health*, the Divine Child devotes itself to achieving the goal of Agape by putting love into action.

Using the Constructive Components to Achieve Radiant Health

The seven steps on *The Journey to Radiant Health* establish a path of awareness and healing that propels you to Radiant Health. The three constructive components will help you: develop a relationship with your Spirit Child, heal childhood wounds, reclaim your childhood dreams, master the ego, break unhealthy habits or behaviors and serve others.

Each constructive component is pertinent to the successful implementation of the seven individual steps. But, one particular component—either focus, commitment or discipline—is especially useful to the implementation of each specific step. As you review the seven steps, the primary constructive component will be defined as the step is outlined. The application of the constructive components to each step assures positive results.

Review of the Seven Steps to Radiant Health

Step 1. Conscious Breathing: Your Foundation

Breath is the gateway to your experiences. Conscious breathing is your foundation on *The Journey to Radiant Health*. In Chapters 4 and 7, you learned how to use conscious breathing to raise your conscious awareness. Commitment and discipline are necessary to establish a consistent conscious breathing practice, but *Focus* will keep your mind engaged in the task of conscious breathing.

Step 2. Put Love into Action: The Essential Practice

Chapter 8 offered the spiritual axiom: *Love is the highest Truth one can put into Action*. Commitment and discipline are essential attributes to put love into action, but *Focus* keeps you mentally clear and centered on expressing the qualities of Love, especially forgiveness, acceptance, compassion and trust. Focus also helps you to express the other heart-based characteristics of Agape that reside in center of the emotional body.

Step 3. Pray and Meditate Every Day: Strengthen Your Contact with the Divine

Chapter 8 also described the power of prayer and meditation. Daily prayer and meditation develops, strengthens and maintains your ability to open your heart and contact and hear messages from your Guides, Angels and Ascended Masters. The power of prayer can facilitate emotional, mental and physical healing. The effects of meditation include reduced stress and tension, lowered blood pressure, feelings of peace and serenity and the opening of your mind to higher levels of conscious information.

Although focus and discipline are important to make a concerted effort to pray and meditate daily, *Commitment* enables you to develop a strong relationship with Love and the Divine. Commitment will help you keep the intentions of your prayer pure and your heart open during meditation.

Step 4. Develop a Relationship with Your Spirit Child: Heal Trauma and Retrieve the Lost Parts of Your Soul

Chapter 17 introduced you to the Spirit Child. Your Spirit Child is the gatekeeper of the heart. The Spirit Child knows all of your traumas and dreams. Establishing a relationship with your Spirit Child is another step in the healing process which eventually leads you to your truth centers. Soul Retrieval heals trauma, and leads to the discarding of unhealthy belief systems, attitudes and perceptions and the adoption of healthy new ones about you and the world around you. Heal the trauma and your heart opens, restoring the flow of your emotional body's creative energy.

Using focus and discipline to make contact with your Spirit Child is important. *Commitment*, however, enables you to develop a strong relationship with your Spirit Child and solidify the healing process that will bring you back to your Divine nature.

Step 5. Be Honest and Truthful in All Your Affairs: Solidify the Connection to Your Heart and Achieve Emotional Maturity

Chapters 24 to 27 described the destructive effects of the ego and fear. The eradication of ego habits and fear is one of the more challenging paths on *The Journey to Radiant Health*. Being honest in all your affairs will enable you to overcome fear and achieve emotional maturity. Focus and commitment are important factors in being honest, but *Discipline* enables you to stay the course of facing your fears and overcoming the tendency to fall back into blatant and subtle patterns of dishonesty.

Step 6. Find Your Life's Purpose: Complete the Process to Retrieve Your Spirit Child's Dreams

A full discussion of how to ascertain your life's purpose has yet to be presented. It can be found in Chapter 33. To get a head start on finding your life's purpose, complete the list that contains your Spirit Child's dreams. The list should contain all the things that brought you joy and that you dreamed of being. Your life's purpose will be found in this list.

Part of your life's purpose is to become a living example of Love. This means mastering the ego and overcoming its obstacles. Although focus and commitment are essential to your search, *Discipline* is the primary constructive component to use to successfully ascertain your life's purpose.

Step 7. Serve Others: Achieve Radiant Health and Experience Lasting Peace and Joy

When you find your life purpose, you will also discover your Divine talents and gifts. These gifts are meant to be used in the spirit of serving others. When you use them to serve the needs of others you will experience great joy and fulfillment and feel a great sense of accomplishment and peace. The seven steps on The Journey to Radiant Health will enable you to be fully present and aware during the journey itself. Because *The Journey to Radiant Health* is the process of learning to be fully present, with yourself and others, in each and every moment of your life, all three components—*Focus, Commitment* and *Discipline*—are essential to the process. The three constructive components will propel you into the present moment, enable you to live in conscious awareness, fully embrace the journey and experience Radiant Health.

The Masculine Constructive Components and the Feminine Truth Centers

The constructive components and the truth centers (see diagram on page 148) occupy the third layer of the mental and emotional bodies respectively. In accordance with the principle of Yin and Yang, when the constructive components and truth centers are brought into communion the result is balance, harmony and synthesis.

When used to support one another, they will take you straight to the heart of truth.

When the synthesis of masculine and feminine energy occurs, your heart and mind open to higher Spiritual perspectives. Thought and emotion merge to move into the heart and produce the highest truth—Love—which becomes the focal point for all your actions.

Use the Constructive Components to Master the Ego

To experience Radiant Health, it is necessary to master the ego personality, and the constructive components are your greatest allies in the quest to meet the challenge. The constructive components enable you to maintain vigilance over the ego and a single point of reference, Love. With your focus, commitment and discipline pinpointed on Love, you can transcend paradigms of fear and overcome ego behaviors. This includes the ego desire to use the components of separation. As the constructive components, focus, commitment and discipline, are fixed on expressing the heart-based qualities of Agape, your ability to exemplify the highest standards of behaviors such as honesty, charity, integrity, patience and non-violence will grow.

Use the Constructive Components
to Raise Your Vibration

You can use the power of the constructive components to raise your frequency, breaking the chains of darkness, ignorance and fear that bind you to the lower frequency of ego thoughts, emotions, behaviors and beliefs. Raising your vibration will extricate you from the destructive cultural and societal patterns that have been imprinted in your ancestral and familial DNA for generations.

On *The Journey to Radiant Health*, it is important to develop a strong ability to maintain focus, commitment and discipline. This will enable you to distance yourself from the reactive, fear-filled thought patterns and emotions that still resonate and reverberate in the collective consciousness.

Until the light fully dissolves the darkness, the fearful vibrations contained in the collective consciousness will remain strong and unyielding. The constructive mental body components will help you break the chains of fear before their force can pull you back into bondage.

Use the Constructive Components to Break the Chains of Fear

It takes time to break the habit of reacting and the constructive components will help you persevere. Commit to the goal of living in the moment and acting from the heart, and you will break the chains that bind you to fear. Every moment will become an opportunity to practice bestowing forgiveness, acceptance and compassion on yourself and others. Eventually you will establish and become rooted in the habit of acting from Love.

Focus, commitment and discipline will now be discussed in detail, with exercises following each section.

FOCUS

Your success on *The Journey to Radiant Health* is determined in large part by your ability to stay focused on step two: putting love into action. Focus is a skill that needs to be developed. When the skill of focus is weak or ineffective, the mind will wander aimlessly, flittering in and out of the endless repository of daydreams and thought forms that arise from the subconscious. Once developed, focus can help you to manifest any goal or intention that you set in your mind.

Focus and Goal-Setting

A clear focus enables you to set a goal and develop a plan of action to achieve that goal. A strong focus will also keep you moving forward when fear, obstacles or distractions threaten to derail your effort.

As you train the mind to focus, your awareness expands. It is said that awareness is responsible for up to 80% of all healing. Develop and strengthen the skill of focus and your awareness will increase to the point where you can quickly identify the ego and release its fears as they arise.

Buddhists claim that conscious breathing is one of the most effective practices to discipline the mind and develop and strengthen focus. Use the exercise below to develop or improve your ability to focus.

EXERCISE:
DEVELOP AND IMPROVE FOCUS

1. Light a candle and place it in front of you.

2. Sit in front of the candle, breathe in and out normally and focus your attention on the candle's flame.

3. Sharpen your focus by keeping your attention on the candle's flame. Notice when your attention wanders away from the candle's flame.

4. When your focus wanes or is distracted, immediately return it to the flame.

5. Each time you practice, make note of how long you are able to keep your focus on the candle flame, and keep track of your progress.

Epilogue to the Focus Exercise

After a few moments of practice, you might notice the mind becomes distracted. Your attention might shift to external sounds such as cars, birds, a passing airplane or an air conditioner. Or your focus might drift to the internal dialogue, coming up with questions such as *"What should I have for lunch?"* or *"Did I leave the bathroom light on?"* The mind can even distract you with pictures of past events or daydreams. These experiences might trigger emotions such as frustration, irritation or impatience.

Each time you catch your mind wandering, return your focus to the flame. The more you practice, the sharper your focus will become. Also, know when to take a break. When you notice that you are consistently losing focus, get some rest or take a break.

Use Focus to Raise Your Vibration

The skill of focus can be used to raise your vibration. When you develop the ability to maintain a fairly keen and consistent focus on your breathing, add the phrase *"Raise my vibration."* Repeat the phrase over and over. With the mind focused on the breath, open your heart and allow it to be filled with love.

As your vibratory rate increases, one of the more palpable effects is a soothing, relaxing and tingling sensation that moves through the body. The sensation sends waves of peace, love and serenity into all three bodies.

Be aware that when you focus on the phrase *"Raise my vibration,"* any deep-seated fears that are imprinted in the cellular structure will rise to the surface. Raising your vibration can start dissolving the lower vibratory patterns of fear lodged in the emotional, mental and physical bodies. When fears arise, it is crucial to identify and express them. Otherwise, the fears will sink back down and reclaim their niche.

As you develop and strengthen the skill of focus, your ability to remain supremely focused on your breath and quiet the internal ego-chatter will become steadfast. Your truth centers, and in particular the heart's truth and wisdom, become fully accessible and will provide you with clear answers to your questions, and clear guidance and direction.

Finally, be cognizant of where you place your focus—whether it be pleasure or pain, limiting beliefs or expansive thoughts, goals or desires, Radiant Health or love—because that is what will likely manifest. When you want to accomplish a task or you are facing challenges, focus on questions that start with how or what, such as *"What actions can be taken to achieve the goal?"* or *"How can this obstacle be overcome?"* "How" and "what" questions focus the mind. They challenge it to come up with empowering answers to move you towards realizing your goals.

COMMITMENT

With the constructive mental body component—focus—in place, commitment is the next component to add to the mix. Commitment establishes the health and vitality of a relationship because it has a tangible effect on your life as well as the lives of others. As such, commitments should not be entered into lightly or taken lightly, regardless of their content or context.

A commitment is a promise to yourself or others to do what you say you will do and be responsible and accountable for your actions. Backing your words with a commitment is a declaration of your intention to do everything in your power to complete the task.

When you commit, you give your word.

On *The Journey to Radiant Health,* your word symbolizes your integrity as well as your commitment to put love into action. The highest commitment on *The Journey to Radiant Health* is to embody the qualities of Agape and put love in action in all your relationships; especially those who challenge your ability to be tolerant, patient, peaceful, detached and balanced.

Commitments can help you break unhealthy habits or establish new ones, build momentum or consistency, work towards a goal or dream, and persevere through the ordinary tasks of an assignment.

Following a commitment to completion can strengthen your character, improve your self-esteem and prove your ability to persevere. Failure to follow through on a commitment can shatter trust, bring on pain or suffering and destroy relationships.

Two Fears Can Stop You from Making Commitments

There are two fears that can stop you from committing to embark on *The Journey to Radiant Health* or any other endeavor: the fear of failure and the fear of success. These fears need to be identified, owned, expressed, and released before you can move forward.

The fear of failure relates to the first core belief behind fear: you are powerless to change. The fear that you will fail needs to be acknowledged, otherwise the possibility exists that you might not follow the commitment to completion. However, failure is not realistic on *The Journey to Radiant Health* because the journey is a lifetime endeavor. Success is not dependent on how well you do or how much you achieve, but rather the effort that you put forth.

On *The Journey to Radiant Health,* success is equal to effort.

It is your effort to practice conscious breathing, heal your wounds, reclaim your dreams and open your heart that enables you to grow. When you grow, you change, and as you change, you will realize that you are not powerless. While your commitment establishes a relationship between you and your dreams, the deeper growth and lesson is not in achieving the goal, but in the experience and savoring of the journey itself.

The fear of success relates to the second core belief behind fear: something you value can be taken from you. The ego can project fear-based beliefs such as the idea that you do not have the education, money, personality or drive to be successful. The deeper underlying fear is that if you succeed it will lead to changes that cause problems, or you will not be able to sustain your success. If everything you work for can ultimately be taken away, then the ego projects its greatest fear and concludes: "*Why bother?*"

Fear can sabotage your effort before you ever take an action.

The subconscious fear of success will stop you from committing to do the things that you feel most passionately about. Again, identify the fear and express it. Then move forward with the awareness that the knowledge gathered from your experiences can never be taken from you.

Commitment, and The Journey to Radiant Health

Make the commitment to put the seven steps on *The Journey to Radiant Health* into practice and you will learn and grow. It does not matter whether you practice the steps perfectly. Just give your best effort and always affirm that you are doing your best.

Every attempt you make to practice conscious breathing, put love into action, pray and meditate, heal your wounds, be honest, open your heart or serve others empowers you a little bit more.

The key is to keep making the effort. Keep focusing on the greater goals: to live in the moment and aspire to exemplify the heart-based qualities of Agape. Your efforts will make a difference in your life and the lives of others. With practice you will grow into a human being who consistently expresses love and truth in action.

DISCIPLINE

Discipline rounds out the Sacred Trinity of constructive components. Discipline arises from the root word *disciple* which is defined as "one who follows or is devoted to a teaching or a course of action."

On *The Journey to Radiant Health*, discipline supports your commitments and enables you to devote time and energy to your life's purpose. The *stick to it* energy inherent in discipline supports your focus and commitments and is key to achieving Radiant Health or any other goal. When ego behaviors such as resistance, procrastination, stubbornness or self-criticism impede your progress or threaten to sabotage your efforts, it is your ability to stay disciplined that will keep you focused and on track, moving towards your goal.

Discipline, the Ego and Goal-Setting

Goal-setting is a great way to achieve a desired outcome, but being goal-oriented is the antithesis of being disciplined. On *The Journey to Radiant Health*, the primary goal—to put love into action—emphasizes creating healthy, loving relationships. When reaching the goal becomes more important than putting love into action and nurturing and honoring your relationships, then the ego drive has taken hold.

When the ego takes control, being *"goal-oriented"* becomes an excuse for escaping life and your relationships. Being able to put love into action means being a human being, not a human doing. Those who become myopic in the pursuit of a goal miss the beauty of the journey and undermine the opportunity to foster healthy relationships.

Be Devoted to What You Love

A disciple follows a course of action because of the love and devotion felt for the course. Devote yourself to that which you love, and the importance of reaching the goal will not matter. Paradoxically, by being immersed in that which you love, the goal will materialize itself. The fruit of your labor will be in your effort, not in the attainment. Taking the time to smell the roses and share the triumphs and pitfalls of the process are part of the journey itself.

Being disciplined in your efforts to stay the course strengthens your character. Your discipline makes it possible to perform the mundane tasks that need to be completed to achieve the goal. Discipline is a call to be devoted, and the highest devotion is to love God and others, because everyone and everything is God, including you.

Use Focus, Commitment and Discipline to Follow Your Life's Purpose and Experience Radiant Health

After you ascertain the Spirit Child's dreams, make a commitment to create a plan of action and use discipline to put your plan into action. If you run into obstacles do not let the ego make excuses or return to its comfort zones. Instead, use the *"how"* and *"what"* questions to find a way to stick with the commitment and complete the task. By integrating discipline with the constructive components, focus and commitment, you will be able to follow your outlined course of action.

Achieving a goal is the process of taking a series of actions, the first of which is to get clear on the goal itself. People often languish in dissatisfaction, not because they lack the talent, ability or power to create change, but because they do not take the time to make a disciplined effort to clarify their dreams or goals.

As you put the seven steps to Radiant Health into action direct your focus, commitment and discipline towards the journey's broader perspective and its foremost precept: *"Love is the highest truth one can put into action."* Rather than being trapped by the ego's desire to achieve a goal, use your discipline to keep your focus on the greater goal of Radiant Health.

FOCUS, COMMITMENT AND DISCIPLINE EXERCISE
PART I

1. Write a daily list of what you want to accomplish. Start with simple things so that you build some *"wins."* Writing a daily list will support your commitment to create new and healthy habits and help you develop greater focus and discipline. With each thing you complete from the list you will gain a greater sense of accomplishment.

2. Transfer whatever has not been accomplished to the next day's list.

3. After you make a commitment, do not break it. For example, if you make a commitment to clean your house on Thursday and a friend calls and asks you to go dancing on Thursday, keep your commitment.

    The only hard and fast rule when you make a commitment is to follow it through. In the course of carrying a commitment to completion, circumstances that are beyond your control will often arise. Be flexible and make adjustments as the situation dictates, but keep your word. The key is to make a habit of following through and carrying out your commitments.

4. Add a challenging goal to your list. It does not have to be an earth-shattering goal, but make it something you want to do but have put off because it brings up fear.

FOCUS, COMMITMENT AND DISCIPLINE
EXERCISE PART II:
CREATE A PLAN OF ACTION

1. Write out a clear and detailed plan of action to carry out your commitment.

   For example, if your commitment is to bring more fun and laughter into your relationship, then your plan of action might include the following steps:
   A- Write out a list of fun activities.
   B- Share the list with your partner.
   C- Set aside some "fun time."
   D- Ask your partner to write out his/her own fun activities.
   E- Try some of your partner's fun ideas.

2. Set time-lines and dates to complete each step in your plan of action. Review your goals every two to four weeks.

3. Be flexible and make adjustments as necessary. If you run into obstacles or your plan does not work, do not give up. Be willing to add new items or restructure your original plan if it needs further clarification.

   For example, be willing to adjust the times you choose as well as who will choose an activity, and from which list will it be picked.

4. As you complete your commitments, make new ones.

FOCUS, COMMITMENT AND DISCIPLINE EXERCISE
PART III:
ESTABLISHING A NEW HABIT

1. Use the steps outlined in Part II as a guideline for this exercise and add the following steps:

2. Write out the reasons for wanting to establish the new habit.

3. In your plan include repetitive actions that will help you form the new habit.

   For example, if you want to get up earlier: buy an alarm clock, go to bed earlier or use a suggestive message when you go to sleep, such as *"I will wake up at seven."* Repeat the message until you fall asleep.

4. Employ the *"buddy system"* to keep your discipline sharp and active.

   Pick a buddy who can support your effort and is non-judgmental and enthusiastic. Set regular times and dates to make your calls. Share your commitments, time-lines for completion, fears, triumphs and overall progress towards your goals.

5. Put your plan into action and use it until the new habit is established.

6. If your discipline wanes during the process, reread your reasons for wanting to form the new habit and use the Passion and the Will exercises to give you a boost.

Passion and Will Support the Constructive Components

In Chapter 12 you learned that anger, expressed from its center, yields two dynamic energies: motivation and determination. These energies can propel you to the completion of a commitment. But, rather than having to get angry and harness its energy, the emotional body element, Passion, and the mental body element, Will, can be used to produce the same dynamic energies.

When used simultaneously, Passion and Will provide a harmonic balance of feminine and masculine energy. Passion kindles your creative energy, motivating you to put the seven steps to Radiant Health into action. Will provides you with the determination to carry them to completion. Passion furnishes inspiration, enthusiasm and excitement and Will contributes drive, perseverance and direction.

Any goal is attainable through dedication and hard work. However, without strong convictions to support your commitment, it is improbable that you will expend the extra energy needed to push beyond the tough challenges. Without Passion or Will to support your commitment, the possibility that you will complete the commitment is poor. Prior to making a commitment be sure that you are able to satisfactorily answer the questions, *"Do I feel passionate about the commitment?"* and *"What do I need to do to complete the commitment?"*

A Final Note on the Constructive Components

In the upcoming physical body section, you will find a chapter that addresses your life's purpose in detail. You can refer back to the exercises in this chapter to assist you to uncover and carry out your life's purpose.

29

The Mental Body Center: Truth and Wisdom

Although truth and wisdom are Spiritual components found in the mental body's center, they originate in the heart. The practice of contemplation—in which quiet time is spent seeking the appraised value of an action before it is taken—allows truth and wisdom to reside in the mental body. Contemplation enables the mind to access the heart's truth center. Balance between the mental and emotional bodies brings truth and wisdom to light.

Use the Heart and Mind to Validate Truth

Because the mind can be influenced by the ego, it is best to validate the truth by harmonizing the mind's aptitude for logic and reasoning with the heart's ability to express Agape. When the light of truth arises from the heart, it always *feels right*, is grounded in love, follows the dictates of common sense and does no harm. Conflict and confusion are never present when truth is spoken or wisdom displayed.

When truth and wisdom are expressed, peace and confidence permeate your consciousness in direct contrast to the intensity or challenge of a situation. The way in which truth is delivered enables it to naturally evolve into its exalted Spiritual form, wisdom. When the desire to seek and follow truth and wisdom becomes paramount in your mind, your words and actions will arise naturally from your heart.

By challenging the mind to contemplate and then embody the highest truths, maturity will take hold. Your ability to discriminate between that which produces Radiant Health or dis-ease will become stronger. Harmful thoughts, words, emotions, behaviors and actions will become unmistakably clear and subconscious fears identified and released. As fears are released, they can be replaced with habits and behaviors grounded in truth and wisdom.

The Journey to Truth and Wisdom

The journey to live in the light of truth and wisdom starts by making a conscious decision to study, contemplate and put into action the teachings of great masters and sages. Contemplate a master's teachings, and the hidden gems of truth and wisdom can be extracted and put into practice. As the teachings are lived, the realization will take place that you are perfect, and people who taught or convinced you otherwise were mistaken.

TRUTH

Truth is always found in the heart. Truth is simple, powered by the tenets of common sense that enable us to live our lives unencumbered by the trappings of the ego and its complexities.

Throughout the ages, enlightened masters have passed down Spiritual principles for living life to the masses. Over time, these Spiritual truths have become the foundation for the world's many religions and Spiritual teachings. Yet, when the teachings of the great masters are examined it will be discovered that, regardless of religious affiliation, all advocate the same values, practices and principles for living a healthy, happy life and achieving self-realization. The only difference is found in their unique methods of expressing universal truths.

For example, Lord Krisna's teachings, found in the Spiritual text the Bhagavad Gita, are studied by Hindus. Moses handed down the Ten Commandments, and the precepts practiced in Judaism are contained in the five books of the Torah. Buddha established the

Four Noble Truths and Eightfold Noble Path, often referred to as the Middle Path, the Spiritual practice of Buddhists. Mohammed received the 114 Suras that are contained in the Quran (Koran), the spiritual text adhered to by Muslims. Lao Tze authored the Tao Te Ching, the classic Spiritual text followed by Taoists. Jesus proclaimed Love to be the highest truth and commanded others to *"Love thy neighbor as thyself."* The teachings and principles of Jesus are contained in the Bible's New Testament.

Putting Spiritual Truths into Action

Each Spiritual doctrine mentioned above contains a formula for living that can arouse you to greater levels of conscious awareness. They contain simple standards for living that can lead you to Radiant Health. And, although they are simple, they are not easy, because rather than being preached a master's Spiritual truths must be put into action.

Being that we are endowed with free will, all Spiritual truths, including those set down by the masters, are subject to individual interpretation. Free will allows even the most virtuous and seemingly incorruptible truths to be compromised for the sake of convenience, or manipulated to fit personal agendas and desires. An individual or teacher might change the precepts and definitions of Spiritual truth to justify or defend his ego actions. The ego can also placate feelings of guilt and shame that plague the mind when an action is in clear conflict with the guiding light of a Spiritual truth.

Living in Truth Creates Freedom

"The truth will set you free" is an adage that speaks to a fundamental ideal on *The Journey to Radiant Health.* The ideal is that by firmly adhering to a set of Spiritual truths, it is possible for you to achieve true freedom. Liberation from all things that enslave you to ego consciousness and cause you to suffer is true freedom. The Spiritual doctrines of the masters can set you free. Contemplate and whole-

heartedly practice the Spiritual principles set forth by the masters and you will be freed from suffering.

To comprehend the deeper truths contained in Spiritual doctrine, contemplate the doctrine. Contemplation enables you to take spoken or written words and extract the truths, avoid misinterpretations and differentiate between the guidance of Spirit and the self-centeredness of ego. The discipline of contemplation enables you to strip the ego chaff from the kernels of Love, so that you can put the heart of truth into action.

Mahatma Gandhi said that truth is like a pie; everyone has his own slice, but nobody has the whole pie. Personal truths are one slice of the pie, and while being important, they are only one of three categories of truth.

The Three Categories of Truth

The first of the three categories, personal truths, is not always in alignment with Spiritual truth because it can arise from the ego. Personal truths are often a product of ideas and beliefs that are colored by personal experience. They are a valid expression of an individual view of truth.

The second category, world truths, is founded on truths that apply in physical reality. World truths are based on the law of physical duality and include phenomena such as the sun rising in the east and setting in the west, there being 24 hours in a day, a north and south pole and two sexes, women and men.

Karma, which is often misconstrued as being something negative, describes the dualistic law of cause and effect, or action and reaction. The law of Karma is analogous to the adage *"As you sow, so shall you reap."* It is interesting to note that while the law of Karma comes from the East, and the adage *"As you sow, so shall you reap"* arises from the West, they both describe the same Spiritual principle of duality and balance that exists in the world, yet they belong to the category of universal truths.

Universal truths are the final category, and are also known as absolute truths. According to the Buddha, one absolute truth is "There is nothing absolute in the world; everything is relative, conditioned and impermanent." Universal truths are established on paradoxical, yet fundamental, unchanging laws as described by the Buddha. Another universal truth is that everything in existence is eternally in a state of flux.

With the disciplined eye of discernment, common threads of love and truth can be discovered among all Spiritual doctrines. When we study all great Spiritual doctrines we will find that the same truths are found in each.

For truth to have a health-producing and healing effect, it is important that it be delivered with love. Love is truth's balancing and complementary counterpart. One way to infuse love into any truthful expression is to express it quietly and with reverence. Regardless of whether it is a universal truth or one grounded in a Spiritual tradition, free will and free choice enable us to reject truth on the spot, regardless of how *spot on* it is.

Conversely, by sharing truth in a mindful, softly spoken, compassionate and humble way, it stands a greater chance of being heard. Respecting and honoring an individual's free will to choose, perceive, think or believe as he or she pleases honors their journey and reduces the odds of becoming embroiled in an emotional argument or fight about whose truth is right. Adhere to this principle of truth and your heart will be sufficiently expanded.

TRUTH EXERCISE

To ascertain the truth in any situation, follow this course of action:

1. Engage the mind in the task of conscious breathing.

2. Use the discipline of contemplation to focus on what has been spoken or written.

3. Access the truth centers and determine whether love is present in the truth and how the truth will serve the greater good.

4. Be patient. Commit to search until you find the love-based answer to your problem or challenge.

WISDOM

Life experiences provide you with a great opportunity to grow wise. It takes time to accrue wisdom, but the process can be accelerated by putting the Spiritual teachings of the masters into action in your life. When you open your heart and embrace all that life has to offer—its pain and joy, its sorrows and laughter, its hard work and play—their teachings and Spiritual truths will be realized. Wisdom is cultivated and matured by a willingness to experience life by putting Spiritual principles into action.

Wisdom is not accrued by intellectual endeavor.

Wisdom is acquired after making a decision to seek the highest truths and then actively committing to practice them in daily routines. To put love into action is one way to gain the kind of experience that transforms into wisdom. This is the most sublime journey you can embrace in life. By practicing the truth of love, you will create plenty of opportunities to gain the experiential knowledge that *all is one*. As you put love into action, your experiences will lead to knowledge, which can then mature into wisdom.

The Path of Wisdom

Embark on the path of wisdom and eventually you will reach the point of Spiritual uplifting that brings about the cessation of suffering. The key is to find the balance between what a teacher imparts, how it resonates in your truth centers and being ready to put the teaching into action. When a profound Spiritual truth is imparted and you are not ready to hear it, you will be unable to act on it and receive its wisdom.

Wisdom is imparted by a great many teachers who freely transmit their Spiritual knowledge to mankind, and yet it can only be heard by those whose hearts are open to receive it. A great many role models and teachers are available to you through study or direct experience. The opportunity to embrace their wisdom is always available to you. The Tibetan Buddhist story below illustrates the wisdom of mastering fundamentals.

The Wisdom of Mastering Fundamentals

A young boy is sent to school by his parents to begin his education. When the boy arrives at school, the teacher writes the number one on a chalkboard and instructs the students to write the number on their paper. After the students practice writing the number one, the teacher asks if they are ready to move on to number two.

The boy does not feel ready to move on.

The teacher gives him more time. By the end of the day the other students have completed the number two, but the boy still feels he has not mastered the number one. During the next three days he works diligently, but has not mastered the number one. As the other students advance, the boy falls further behind. Now impatient with his lack of progress, the teacher encourages him to skip the number one and just move on.

The boy cannot.

After two weeks, the teacher takes the boy to his parents and explains that the boy is not a capable student. The boy, feeling that he has disgraced his family and himself, says, *"I must go away and not return until I have learned the lesson."*

Years later the young man returns to the teacher's classroom. *"Sir,"* he says to the teacher, *"many years ago I had to go away because I could not master the number one. I now believe that I understand the lesson."* The teacher, remembering the student, says, *"Then demonstrate your knowledge."* The young man walks over to the chalkboard and as he writes the number one on it, to the teacher's astonishment, the chalkboard splits in two.

The Wisdom in Parables

By repetition, the young man literally and experientially learned the power of the number one, but this is not the story's only message. Mythological tales, parables and anecdotes contain dimensions that challenge us to dig deeper to extract a story's hidden pearls of wisdom. For example, beneath the surface of this tale's conflict is a story of triumph that chronicles a boy's growth, humility, courage, commitment, perseverance, love, discipline, focus, honor, passion and honesty.

Spiritual and mythological tales are steeped in wisdom that you can glean by putting the teachings into action. Wisdom can be found on many paths. However, walking the paths that challenge you to master the fundamentals in life bestows the greatest wisdom.

A Zen adage states, *"Before enlightenment, chop wood, carry water; after enlightenment, chop wood, carry water."* There is great wisdom in this saying, but it cannot be known without a sincere desire to contemplate its deeper meaning. The nature of wisdom is not found in being quick, but rather in being slow and methodical, and following the footsteps and principles of the masters. Sow seeds of consistency, contemplation, introspection and perseverance and you will reap a harvest of happiness, bliss and contentment.

Buddhists say, *"Enlightenment is granting freedom to everything around you."* Wisdom dictates that when you are suffering, you need only find your attachment to find its roots. Cut the attachment and release it to restore your peace of mind and joy.

Wisdom can be found in the heart of every culture known to mankind. It is slow to stir, for wisdom only emerges when all things have been taken into consideration. This section closes with one of the most common and yet greatest expressions of wisdom. Give it careful consideration before you take any action.

We are one.

SECTION SIX

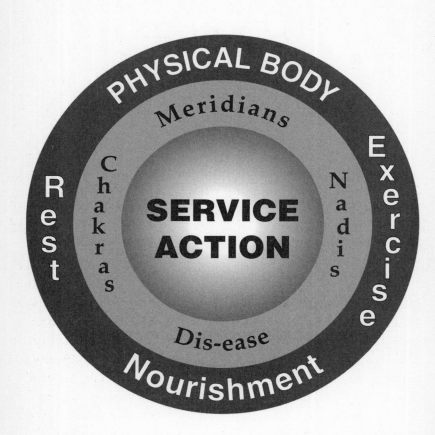

Color chart available at:
www.radiantkeys.com

30

The Physical Body

Tune your frequency to one vibration,
the vibration of the Divine, and let all others go.
—Babaji

The physical body represents the merging of the emotional and mental bodies, the heart and mind, and masculine and feminine energy. It is the transcendence of duality that places the physical body at the crown of The Sacred Trinity of Radiant Health (see page 60). The resulting state of wholeness leads to the emergence of the Divine Child.

The Divine Child is the synthesis of masculine/mental body energy and feminine/emotional body energy. The Divine Child transcends the ego, rises above limitations (including those imposed by duality) and exists in pure and unchanging conscious awareness. It exists beyond the Cartesian split between God and humanity, science and Spirit, and mind and body. Aware of its divinity, purity and perfection, the Divine Child effortlessly slides the scale between its feminine and masculine energies, deftly harmonizing the two. The Divine Child's ability to transcend the illusion of separation enables it to actualize Agape in every moment, intention and action.

The Divine Child

The Divine Child is supremely flexible, adapting to the movement and flow of any interaction, event or circumstance. Its actions always arise from the heart of pure awareness, and it has the strength and confidence to trust and follow its own Divine guidance, especially when the message opposes protocol or etiquette or is contrary to what appears to be the right action.

The Divine Child flows through life with innocence and reverence, in awe of everything in the world including the magic and mystery that defines life. It exists only in the present moment because it is free from attachments and emotional charges like judgments, prejudices and resentments.

Fear and worry do not trap the Divine Child. It knows that everything is in perfect order and trusts that the greater purpose will reveal itself, even when things do not go its way, or it does not understand the meaning of an event.

The Physical Body Is Your Sacred and Divine Temple

The physical body is generally identified as who you are, but it is not. Instead, the physical body is your sacred temple and the home to the Divine Child. The Divine Child is your Spirit. Although Spirit cannot be seen or touched, when your masculine and feminine energies are synthesized, your true nature, Spirit, is awakened and manifests as loving actions. The physical body expresses this awakening as Radiant Health.

The moments or periods in your life when you flow with grace and ease, and are free from stress and worry, mark the times when the Divine Child is being expressed through you. It is during these times that you experience Radiant Health. The greater your commitment to practice conscious breathing, the greater your potential to live in full conscious awareness and become the Divine Child.

In the three bodies, the physical body acts as the last warning line of defense. Unresolved emotional or mental issues block the free flow of energy through the physical body, causing the heart to close and the Divine Child to recede. Physical dis-ease lets you know that disintegration has occurred. It affords you an opportunity to grow in awareness and take measures to heal.

The Physical Body Is a Reflection of Your Thoughts, Emotions and Experiences

Your physical body contains an energetic imprint of every emotion, thought and experience you have ever had. It also is a reflection of what you put into it. Your physical posture reflects your attitudes, perceptions and beliefs. How you treat your body speaks volumes about how you feel about yourself.

When you feel confident and joyful you stand tall with your shoulders straight and chin up. When you feel depressed or insecure you hunch over, dropping the chin and shoulders. This also works in reverse: the more you slouch, the more depressed or insecure you will feel; the straighter you stand, the more confident and joyful you will feel.

The body functions at its optimum level when: love for God fills your mind and heart, love is expressed by your thoughts and emotions, you eat pure foods and get proper amounts of rest and exercise. You will have as much energy as you need; there will be no limits to what you can accomplish, and you will experience Radiant Health.

Your Most Important Relationship

As your Divine temple, the physical body is your most important relationship. It starts at the moment of birth and continues up to the moment that you take your last breath. No relationship lasts as long—not the one you have with your parents, siblings, friends or lovers. You only get one body to carry you through this lifetime. By exploring the physical body's components and how they affect your holistic health and well-being you can learn how to keep it healthy. It is much easier to experience peace and contentment when the body is healthy and filled with vital life-force energy. Love, nurture and respect the body, and it will function optimally and be a wonderful home.

The Outer Layer of the Physical Body

Radiant physical health is a result of keeping the three fundamental elements of the physical body—nourishment, rest and exercise—in balance. It is well documented that proper nourishment, rest and exercise support optimum physical health. Further, the relationship between the fundamental physical body components and their effects on mental and emotional health are profound. Maintain the balance between each of these elements and you are well on your way to the experience of Radiant Health.

Nourishment

Nutrition describes the utilization of food or substances to produce physical energy, while the word *nourishment* represents a holistic paradigm in which food and substances are used to nurture, heal and maintain the health of each of the three bodies. Nourishment is an important and essential component to the maintenance of physical health and eradication of dis-ease.

A healthy nourishment regimen will help you alter the physical environment from one that invites and supports dis-ease to one that encourages healthy cell and tissue growth, repair and regeneration. But just as important, a healthy nourishment regimen has a potent effect in producing emotional and mental health and well-being.

Using Food to Nourish the Three Bodies

Healthy eating habits create positive change at the cellular and molecular level. The emotional, mental and physical effects of your eating habits can be ascertained by looking at what and where you eat, where you buy your food and how you prepare it.

There are literally thousands of books filled with facts, opinions, theories and a wide variety of scientific information about healthy nutrition. The question of what constitutes healthy nutrition has become so complex that it can be overwhelming and virtually impossible to find two experts who can agree on a simple set of standards that establish a healthy diet.

But a simple paradigm does exist.

In the East, an ancient paradigm exists that assigns an energetic value to foods and substances based on how they affect the three bodies. In the West, a scientific model exists that closely mirrors the Eastern paradigm. Although the Western paradigm does not include the ramifications of foods and substances on the emotional and mental bodies, it still is a valid and complementary system. Study their similarities and you can create a simple set of healthy nourishment standards that limit or eradicate the foods and substances that lead to dis-ease.

The Eastern Paradigm for Healthy Nourishment

The belief that foods can and do affect your emotional and mental health and well-being marks a major difference between Eastern and Western schools of thought on nutrition. Western scientific thought supports dissection, viewing each body separately as if each body is independent and could actually exist apart from the other two. Eastern Spiritual thought supports integration, viewing each body as being entirely interwoven and wholly interdependent with one another. Put them together and the two strike a beautiful balance. Dissection allows for a full examination of the workings of each body, while integration affirms and honors the intrinsic union of all three.

The Eastern paradigm of nourishment is founded on the understanding that food has a holistic effect on an individual. This understanding leads to a paradigm that contains guidelines designed to ensure holistic, rather than individual, nourishment of the three bodies. The Eastern paradigm of nourishment considers the quality of energy in food to be of primary importance in the quest to achieve Radiant Health.

THE THREE GUNAS

The Eastern paradigm of nourishment is based on the three Gunas: the three distinct qualities of energy found in everything in physical reality. The three Gunas are Sattva, which represents purity and knowledge, Rajas, which represents activity and motion, and Tamas, which represents inertia and destruction. In the Eastern paradigm, foods that are enticing and sensual to the palate lose their nourishing value if they disturb any of the three bodies. The study of the three Gunas, as they relate to food, will help you understand the nourishing or destructive effects that specific foods, substances and eating habits have on your emotional, mental and physical health and well-being.

Sattvic Foods

The first category is comprised of sattvic foods, which have a completely positive effect on the three bodies. Sattvic foods include fresh fruit and vegetables, legumes, pure fruit juices, rice, nuts, sprouted seeds, honey, wholemeal breads and herbal teas.

Sattvic foods promote peace and calm. They enhance creative energy, help you maintain your poise and emotional center, and protect you from being easily upset in stressful situations. Sattvic food keeps the mental body clear, alert and focused, and support positive thought forms and an expansive, open mind. Sattvic foods provide vital life force and active energy to the physical body. They help sustain the smooth, effective and efficient function of the muscles, tissues, nerves and internal organs.

Rajasic Foods and Substances

Rajasic foods and substances upset the delicate energetic balance between the three bodies. Rajasic items include coffee, black tea, fish, eggs, salt, chocolate and foods that are too hot, bitter, sour, dry or salty. Consumed in excess, rajasic items provoke intense emotions including frustration, worry and anxiety. They cause excessive stimulation in the physical body, which leads to muscular stress, tension and injury. Rajasic items agitate the mind, making it restless and uncontrollable while provoking ego behaviors such as blame, envy, greed, worry and deceit. Eating too fast also is considered rajasic.

Tamasic Foods and Substances

Tamasic foods and substances rob the body of prana and promote disease. Tamasic items include tobacco, alcohol, drugs, refined sugars, white flour, sharp spices, meat, onions, vinegar, and stale, fermented or overripe foods. Tamasic foods and substances can cause you to lose your emotional equilibrium and mental powers of reasoning. In addition, they can cause you to justify dark, vengeful and destructive behaviors. Intense ego and dis-ease-producing emotions such as depression, anger, greed, lust and rage can be experienced as a result of ingesting tamasic foods and substances. Overeating, which dulls the senses, is considered tamasic. Processed and canned foods are considered tamasic because their prana has been stripped away.

Western Paradigms for Healthy Nourishment

In 1956, the Department of Agriculture developed a plan to address nutritional needs. Its initial dietary guidelines consisted of four basic food groups: (1) meats and dairy products, (2) breads and cereals, (3) fruits and (4) vegetables.

For many years the original guidelines were considered to be the foundation for healthy nutrition. But after years of scientific research that idea changed. A number of disturbing dis-ease trends emerged indicating conclusively that a "balanced diet" consisting of the four food groups led to increased rates of heart disease and cancers.[1] The dis-eases were attributed to high levels of animal fat from meat and dairy products and low levels of dietary fiber: a result of not eating enough fruits and vegetables.

The Food Guide Pyramid

A revised edition was created and is now entitled the *Food Guide Pyramid.* The pyramid is displayed on the following page. The foods contained in the pyramid, when eaten in the suggested proportions, are said to be the foundation of a healthy diet. The bottom of the pyramid contains the foods that lead to optimum physical health, while the top of the pyramid contains the foods to limit or avoid altogether.

The new model is closer to a paradigm for healthy nourishment, but is still incomplete. Former Surgeon General C. Everett Koop proclaimed that poor diet has a significant relationship to dis-ease. He also made the now famous recommendation that we eat a minimum of five servings each of fruits and vegetables a day.[2]

Calories and Caloric Intake

In the Western paradigm, foods are categorized by the measurable amount of heat or energy they produce. One unit of energy is called a calorie. In the Western paradigm of nutrition, caloric intake plays an important part in the maintenance of health. The number of calories an adult requires on a daily basis is determined by factors such as age, weight and level of activity. The typical requirement for an average adult is 3,000 calories per day.

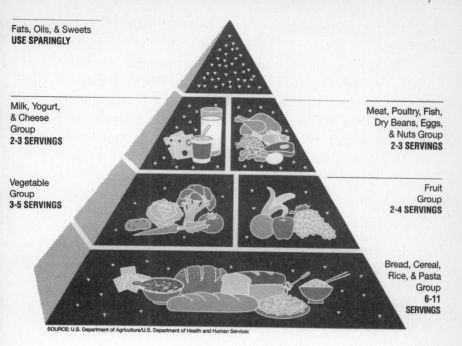

Fats, Oils, & Sweets
USE SPARINGLY

Milk, Yogurt,
& Cheese
Group
2-3 SERVINGS

Meat, Poultry, Fish,
Dry Beans, Eggs,
& Nuts Group
2-3 SERVINGS

Vegetable
Group
3-5 SERVINGS

Fruit
Group
2-4 SERVINGS

Bread, Cereal,
Rice, & Pasta
Group
**6-11
SERVINGS**

SOURCE: U.S. Department of Agriculture/U.S. Department of Health and Human Services

The three elements that provide calories are: carbohydrates, proteins and fats. To maintain physical health it is necessary to eat a combination of foods that contain carbohydrates, proteins and fats in proper proportions. But experts do not often agree on what constitutes proper proportions, and keeping a daily record of calories, carbohydrates, proteins and fats can be cumbersome. Also, while calories can sustain physical health, they do not address the effects of specific foods on your emotional and mental well-being.

The Relationship between pH and Radiant Health

Fortunately, the body's biochemical constituent, pH, constitutes a scientific model that closely follows the Eastern paradigm, and supports the holistic health of the three bodies. pH describes the acid/alkaline level found in the body's tissues and organs as well as the blood.

With the focus on finding a balanced, integrative approach to health, the body's two pH components—acid and alkaline—can be used to create a platform for healthy meals. A fundamental understanding of the body's pH, how it works and the foods that have a positive or negative effect upon it can empower you to eat in a way that facilitates holistic health and greatly reduces the possibility of serious physical dis-ease.

Understanding the Acid/Alkaline Balance

The body produces acid as a by-product of normal metabolism. The body itself is acid in nature. The body does not produce alkaline. Instead, alkaline is introduced to the body by specific foods.

Every food or substance you ingest is categorized as either acid or alkaline based, because when the body digests it, it is reduced to either an acid or alkaline ash. Biochemical research has determined that dis-ease cannot live in an alkaline milieu, but can grow and flourish in an acid environment. By eating foods high in the production of alkaline ash, the body maintains its structural cellular integrity. The ratio of alkaline-based to acid-based foods necessary to maintain healthy, dis-ease-free cells, organs and tissues is 80% alkaline to 20% acid. Sadly, the typical Western diet produces exactly the opposite numbers, 80% acid to 20% alkaline.[3]

This is a frightening statistic when you consider that a highly preventable dis-ease like cancer (which now afflicts one out of every three Americans) flourishes in an acid environment.

Acid Overload: A Recipe for Physical Dis-ease

Here is an illustration of how dis-ease manifests in relationship to your body's acid/alkaline pH. Blood is the principal element that feeds your cells, tissues and organs. Food is the principal element that feeds blood. Acid is introduced to the blood by poor diet.

A critical emotional factor is uncontrolled anger.

Uncontrolled anger causes acid to be dumped into the blood by way of the liver. Acid is filtered out of the blood by the liver and kidneys. However, when poor diet or uncontrolled anger is habitual, the liver and kidneys grow weaker and cannot purge the acid overload in the blood. The blood must rid itself of acid to perform its job, so it dumps the excess acid into the body's organs and tissues. As acid accumulates in the body's tissues and organs, the perfect environment is established for the incubation of dis-ease. To stop this scenario from being played out, take a good look at the foods and substances you are putting into your body.

Change your eating habits and you will change your blood.

It will take time, but ultimately your entire system can be transformed from one in which dis-ease can grow and flourish to one that promotes healthy cells and tissues. Maintain an alkaline pH and you can rid the body of disease and achieve radiant physical health. Dr. Airola states that, *"The higher the ratio of alkaline elements in the diet, the faster the recovery."*[4]

Shifting Your pH from Acid to Alkaline

To start the process of shifting your body's pH from acid to alkaline, choose foods from the alkaline foods list on the following page. The list starts with the highest alkaline-content foods and moves to the lowest. Below the alkaline list you will find a list of acid foods and substances. Acid foods should be taken sparingly and acid substances avoided altogether if possible. The acid list starts with the highest acid-content foods and substances and moves to the lowest.

You can also purchase pH strips at your local drug or health food store and measure your pH. Each morning before you eat, spit into a cup and saturate a small strip of pH paper with the saliva. The color of the pH strip will indicate your pH level. Do not expect your pH to change overnight. Depending on your eating habits, it might take some time for the body to expel the accumulated build-up of acid in the tissues. Make it a point to eat a ratio of 80% alkaline foods to 20% acid foods and the body's pH will eventually shift from acid to alkaline.

Alkaline-Forming Foods

Figs, Blueberries, Prunes, Soybean, Lima beans, Apricots, Spinach, Turnips, Beet greens, Raisins, Almonds, Carrots, Dates, Celery, Cucumber, Cantaloupe, Honeydew, Lettuce, Watercress, Potatoes, Oranges, Pineapple, Grapefruit, Peaches, Apples, Grapes, Bananas, Watermelon, Millet, Brazil nuts, Coconuts and Buckwheat

- Except for millet and buckwheat, most grains are acid-forming.

- Sprouting seeds and grains cause them to become more alkaline.

- All vegetables are highly alkaline.

- To get the most live energy out of juices, drink them fresh, as soon as they are juiced. Include the vegetable tops, and the highest alkaline juices are carrot, beet and celery. All vegetable juices are highly alkaline as are fig and black cherry juice.

- Vegetable juices are preferable to fruit juices because of a lower sugar content.

- Vegetables from the crucifer family such as broccoli, cauliflower, Brussels sprouts, rutabaga, mustard greens and collard greens contain a powerful anti-carcinogenic agent.

- Fresh picked sattvic/alkaline foods are rich in enzymes. Enzymes are the catalysts that supply the metabolic energy for all biochemical reactions that sustain life. They also have the greatest content of pranic life-force energy. Eat them raw or lightly steamed to retain the potency of the enzymes.

Acid-Forming Foods and Substances

Tobacco, Drugs/Medications, Alcohol, Salt, Coffee, Black tea, Food preservatives and additives, Fried meats, Spices, Red meats, Condiments, Fried pastries, Fried fruits/vegetables, White meats, Whole grains, Refined sugar, Dairy products/eggs and Overcooked fruits/vegetables.

Seven Actions to Guard Your Health When You Eat

1. *Never eat when upset.* Your body's biochemistry is affected when you are upset. Eating when upset can lead to digestive problems and other dis-eases.

2. *Pray before you eat your food to raise its vibration.* Before you eat, offer a prayer of thanks and praise to the Creator and Mother Earth for your meals. Prayer will raise the vibration of your food ensuring that your meal emits a nourishing energy.

3. *Eat slowly and chew thoroughly.* As you masticate your food, the mouth releases amylase. This important enzyme starts the digestive process, creating less work for the stomach.

4. *Eat in silence.* Focus on extracting the prana (life-force energy) contained in the food. If you do talk during meals, always keep the topic of conversation light, cheerful and full of laughter. Stay away from intense emotional topics.

5. *Eat with a grateful heart.* Be thankful for the loving relationships, home and other gifts you have. Honor the cycle of life that makes your every meal possible.

6. *Eat only to nourish the body temple.* Do not eat when you feel bored, lonely, dissatisfied or emotionally empty. Work to resolve your unhealthy thoughts and emotions so you will not use food to hide your feelings.

7. *Eat in a pleasant environment.* Eating your meals in an environment that is visually, audibly and sensually pleasing creates a feeling of comfort and relaxation that allows for ease in digestion.

Final Notes on Nourishment

The three Gunas parallel pH. Sattvic foods are alkaline in nature. Tamasic and ragasic foods and substances are acid in nature. The two paradigms (Gunas and pH) illustrate that the balance between East and West, science and Spirit, heart and mind can be found if you seek it.

Although the dietary guidelines from the East and West come from different perspectives, by blending the Gunas and pH you can compose a diet that will nourish the three bodies by increasing your vital physical energy, keeping you mentally alert, emotionally centered and free of dis-ease.

The ancient Chinese proverb *"Moderation in all things keeps one healthy"* sums up nourishment as it relates to Radiant Health. Be moderate in your consumption when ingesting rajasic or tamasic acid-based items. The proverb applies to sattvic foods as well, because ingesting too much of a good thing can also create dis-ease. Minimize your consumption of "fast foods," processed and refined foods, as well as foods that contain additives, preservatives, herbicides and pesticides. Also, follow this simple rule: *If you can't pronounce an ingredient on a food label, do not eat it.*

To simplify your decision-making process about what and how to eat: quiet the mind, tap into your heart and trust your inner guidance. The heart will lead you to the foods that will support your health and nourish each of your three bodies.

WATER

No discussion of nourishment would be complete without the inclusion of water. Second to breath, water is the most nourishing element that can be supplied to the body. Although water contains no calories, it is essential to health and vitality. Consider that Earth is covered by almost 75% water and your body is comprised of up to 80% water, and it is easy to understand that the most important substances you can provide to the body are oxygen and water.

Read This before You Start Drinking

Doctors generally recommend that you drink eight to ten 8-ounce glasses of water a day. But before you gulp all that water, consider that flooding the body with water can overtax the kidneys and bladder and lower your energy levels. Drink slowly and consciously. Also, consider eating water-rich foods such as vegetables, fruits and sprouted seeds to supply the body with that much-needed water.

The higher the ratio of water to non-water foods, the greater the water content in your body. A radiantly healthy ratio is 70% water-rich foods to 30% non-water foods. Note: non-water foods include meats, fish, nuts, legumes, sweets, dairy products and grains. Listen to and trust your body's messages. Stay in tune with your Instinct truth center and you will know when you need to hydrate the body.

Keep Your Body Hydrated

Keeping the body hydrated enables it to expel the toxic waste produced by the body's organs, tissues and cells. If your body's water content is low, it will be unable to remove toxins from its own cells. When the toxic excretions expelled by the cells, tissues and organs are not carried off by the lymphatic system, they are reabsorbed into the system.

Heavy labor, exercise and other sweat-producing activities require more than water to re-hydrate the body. Instead of grabbing an artificially sweetened drink, add a pinch of sea salt and a squeeze of fresh lemon juice to your water, and you will replenish the essential minerals and electrolytes lost during these activities. There is not a substance known to humans that dissolves as many elements as water, and this includes the toxins that result from bodily functions. Also, when the body is properly hydrated the eliminatory organs—kidneys, liver, digestive system, lungs and skin—will all function with greater efficiency.

Make Sure That What You Are Drinking Is Water

Consider your water source. Basic tap water can contain toxic metals and chemicals such as fluoride, chlorine, mercury, lead, ammonia, arsenic, cadmium, chromium and nickel. Toxic metal and chemicals can be removed from tap water by using a reverse osmosis filtration system. You can also place water in a glass container and set it out in the sun for eight hours. The sun is known to destroy micro-bacteria. Also, make sure the pH level of the water is alkaline. Due to pollution and chemical treatment, most water has an acid pH level. To bring your water to a healthy alkaline state, add an alkaline booster, which you can purchase in most health food stores.

FASTING

Fasting dates back thousands of years. Masters such as Jesus, Krisna and Buddha used the practice of fasting as a method to purify the emotional, mental and physical bodies. The purifying process of fasting enables one to gain greater Spiritual clarity and insight. Sages and Yogis engage in fasts regularly to gain Spiritual insights, guidance and direction.

In medical and scientific circles, fasting is widely viewed as a strictly religious or Spiritual practice. Many scientists and medical doctors also consider fasting to be harmful, believing it has no practical medical or health-producing effects. Fasting does in fact have the potential to be dangerous when approached with a flippant attitude.

However, when a specific directive exists for its use, fasting can produce amazing health-producing results. Because the founding principles, process and practice of fasting encompass purification, it should be approached with reverence and respect.

To get the most from a fast, it is important to set a specific intention or purpose and seek professional supervision. Many people safely undertake the kind of long-term fasts that scientific theory claims would cause death, yet they do not die. A clear intention and knowledge of how to fast properly helps, as does the ability to support the body's life force by extracting the prana found in juices, water or particles of air.

On *The Journey to Radiant Health,* fasting can be used to purify the three bodies. It enhances your overall health and well-being and promotes Spiritual clarity and insight.

The Effects of Fasting

Short-term fasts can greatly aid in purifying the physical body because they give the digestive and eliminatory organs a chance to rest. Fasts of a longer duration have been known to rid the body of chronic ailments and deadly dis-eases. During a fast, the energy normally needed to complete the digestive process is transferred to other internal organs and body tissues that need to clear long-standing toxins from them. This purification process promotes a deeper and more complete physical body healing. Fasting also empties you on all levels. It causes you to feel lighter: physically by detoxifying the body, mentally by clearing or eliminating negative thought forms from the mind and emotionally by purifying the heart of toxic emotions.

Choosing Your First Fast: The Master Cleanser

There are many different types of fasts. If you have never fasted and want to start, a 24-hour fast is a good initiation to the fasting experience. You might want to try the fast on your day off from work. Before fasting, set an intention to slow down. Do not overexert yourself physically, mentally or emotionally during your fast.

For your first fast, consider the popular *Master Cleanser.*[5] This fasting recipe uses lemon as an astringent for the tissues and to provide ascorbic acid (vitamin C). Pure maple syrup provides calories for energy, and African cayenne pepper keeps the body warm, purifies the blood and relieves the headaches that sometimes occur due to the detoxification of the body's tissues.

The Master Cleanser formula is simple.

Take one 8-ounce glass of water. Add 1–2 tablespoons pure grade maple syrup, 2 tablespoons lemon juice and 1/10 teaspoon African cayenne pepper. Drink from 6–12 glasses during the day and evening. If the cayenne irritates your throat, you can encapsulate it and take 1 capsule with each 8-ounce glass of water. Notice how your body responds. If you feel overly nauseous, dizzy or weak, discontinue the fast and seek professional guidance. If you feel healthy, stable and strong, you can extend your fast for a period of up to 72 hours.

A Seven-Day Fast

A seven-day fast represents a complete one-week cycle. To embark on a seven-day fast, again set your intention. Use the Master Cleanser and consider including fresh fruit or vegetable juices in your fast. Spinach, carrot, celery and cucumber are a popular and nutrient-rich vegetable combination. You can also juice apples, ginger and carrots, strawberries and watermelons, or other combinations that appeal to you. Juice and drink water as needed.

Longer fasts have been reported to heal chronic ailments. However, any fast that lasts longer than seven days should be performed under the direct supervision of a trained healthcare professional who is experienced in administering long term fasts. Doctors of Ayurvedic, Naturopathy, Homeopathy and Acupuncture are usually skilled and knowledgeable when it comes to fasting. Some M.D.s also support fasting.

Fasting Protocol

As your body expels toxins you might experience headaches, body aches, slight weakness or dizziness. Slow down and take it easy when fasting. Light exercises such as walking or stretching are good, but refrain from strenuous activity. Meditation and Yoga are excellent complementary practices to fasting. In many cultures fasting is considered a Spiritual activity that cleanses the mental and emotional bodies as well as the physical body. The Spiritual clarity and wisdom one can attain during a fast is exponential when compared to non-fasting periods, but is still proportional to the amount of time one takes to turn inward and quietly reflect on one's own life and purpose. Always consult a healthcare professional before fasting.

REST

Rest replenishes your vital energy. During sleep your pranic reserves repair any damage to the body. Inadequate or excessive amounts of sleep can leave you feeling groggy, irritable and energy-deficient. This robs you of your ability to concentrate. Sleep deprivation ultimately leads to accidents and confusion. Sleep is important, but it is only one facet of rest. Engaging in joyful activities that regenerate your vital energy produces the other facet known as "true rest."

Recreation and Its Relationship to Rest

Recreation is rarely considered to be a form of rest. Yet by being an outlet for your creative expression, it reduces stress and tension, replenishing your vital energy. Any truly enjoyable activity, whether it is singing, dancing, drawing or just taking a walk in the park, regenerates your vital life-force energy. Recreation calms the emotions, quiets the mind and reduces stress and tension. When you retire after engaging in a recreative activity, you are likely to get a deeper, more restful night's sleep.

Rest and Its Relationship to the Seasons

Earth's seasonal cycles also affect your need for rest, as do your personal cycles. The spring and summer seasons, being warmer, generate more active energy. During these seasons, you will generally need less rest. The fall and winter seasons, being colder, decrease your active energy. During these seasons, you will generally need more rest.

Energy peaks and valleys also occur during the course of each day and during each season. Forcing yourself to push out of the valleys is unproductive. Forcing yourself to work hard when you need rest is like using a dull saw to cut wood; it wastes energy and can lead to accidents or injuries. Honoring the body's need for rest while in the energy valleys regenerates your energy and sharpens focus and concentration. The results are increased productivity or cutting more wood in less time.

Conscious Breathing Can Reduce the Need for Rest

Conscious breathing increases the prana in the body and can reduce your need for sleep or rest. When used in conjunction with meditation, the prana received by way of conscious breathing can boost your energy. The rest replenisher below is a rejuvenating 15-minute pick-me-up meditation. Although it is not meant to take the place of sleep, its benefits are comparable to a one-hour nap.

REST REPLENISHER MEDITATION

1. Play a 15-minute tape with harmonic overtones, flutes, gongs or gentle nature sounds.

2. Lie down on your back. Legs straight out. Feet slightly spread apart. Arms extended down the side of the body. Make sure that you are comfortable. Put a pillow under your head, knees or lower back if needed.

3. Begin conscious breathing, and focus on drawing in prana on the inhale and completely relaxing the body on the exhale.

4. When the tape ends, as you return to full awareness, gently move your body and then return to your activity.

EXERCISE

Recently, a number of trendy exercises such as Pilates, aerobics, jazzercise and spinning have vaulted to the forefront of the health craze; while traditional exercises such as running, weight training, swimming and biking remain as popular as ever. Exercise provides an outlet for your physical energy, while improving your strength and stamina. But few exercises, if any, were designed to engage the emotional, mental and physical bodies to facilitate holistic health.

Yoga: The Ultimate Workout to Integrate the Emotional, Mental and Physical Bodies

A holistic exercise program is one that takes the three bodies into consideration. Holistic exercise should open the body's subtle energy channels, restore and improve emotional flexibility and balance and increase mental strength and stamina. All of this is in addition to facilitating physical health and well-being.

It is said that a healthy body is a reflection of a healthy mind.

On *The Journey to Radiant Health,* the purpose of exercise is to raise your awareness and work towards the realization that you are Spirit in human form. A holistic discipline is required to meet this criterion. But does one exist?

Although the disciplines of Tai Chi and the Eastern martial arts focus on being aware of and caring for every aspect of your being, there is an ancient Spiritual discipline whose primary focus is to help you achieve self-realization. In the process, it will improve your emotional, mental and physical strength, stamina and flexibility. The Spiritual discipline is Yoga and, by its practice, you can achieve all this and more.

Yoga: An Ancient Spiritual Discipline

In the West, Yoga has become popularized as an exercise, and is considered a great workout. Or, Yoga is often thought of as a series of contortions. Yoga is none of these. Although Yoga was not developed as an exercise, one of its many by-products is that it can offer a great workout to those that practice its postures.

The Spiritual discipline of Yoga was received by way of meditation thousands of years ago by Sages and Rishis in India. The word *Yoga* means "Union with God." As a Spiritual discipline, Yoga is defined in the ancient Sanskrit language as *"Yoga Citham Vriti Norodaha,"* which translates as *"the process of cleansing the movements that arise from the subconscious."*

The Spiritual discipline of Yoga consists of over one hundred parts, including five points, three bodies, seven stages and four paths—one of which contains eight limbs that incorporate a multitude of subsets. However, the Yoga that is familiar to most people in the West consists of three components: *Pranayama, Meditation* and *Asana*. When brought together, the three aspects create a pathway from which one can begin the practice to clear the subconscious.

Each component within the three-pronged discipline contains hundreds and thousands of subset practices. For example, it is said that there are 8,400,000 Asanas, and innumerable Meditations and Pranayamas.

The Three Basic Components of Yoga

The first component: Pranayamas are the breathing exercises of Yoga. Pranayamas, which include conscious breathing and Kriyas—purification techniques—enable you to quiet the mind, develop greater focus and concentration, bring greater amounts of prana into the cells, fill the body with more oxygen, cleanse the circulatory system and access higher levels of conscious awareness.

The second component: Meditation is the discipline of Yoga that enables you to experientially realize the Divine, true self. The discipline of Meditation and its associated practices help you identify the ego and detach from it, and open your heart to receive Spiritual guidance and answers to your questions.

The third component: Asanas are the movements of Yoga. Asanas were developed specifically to cleanse the Nadis and Chakras—the points and intersecting wheels found in the subtle energy astral body. Hatha Yoga—a practice that emphasizes Asanas—prepares the body to sit in meditation for long periods of time. When practiced in conjunction with Pranayama and a meditative state of mind, Asanas can reduce stress and tension, alleviate pain and facilitate healing by dissolving the subtle energy blockages that exist in the astral and physical bodies.

The word *Asana*, when translated, means "posture" or "pose." When engaging in a Yogic Asana practice the primary focus is to perform each movement with a quiet mind, fluid rhythmic breathing pattern and the ability to maintain the pose without struggle, as if you were sitting in rest. The moment an Asana becomes uncomfortable it produces stress and tension, and is no longer considered an Asana. Asanas stimulate, activate and rejuvenate the muscles, tissues, internal organs, blood and lymphatic systems. Contrary to a conventional exercise program, a traditional Asana practice does not emphasize improving the cardiovascular system, flexibility, strength, stamina or balance. Such benefits are simply a by-product of the practice. When Asanas are practiced consistently, you are likely to experience improvements in all these areas.

Yoga Restores Subtle Energy Flow to the Three Bodies

At the core level, the Asanas were developed to dissolve blockages and open and restore the free flow of energy in the astral body's subtle energy systems—Nadis, Meridians and Chakras.

The Nadis, Meridians and Chakras are the points, lines and wheels of energy, respectively, that compose the subtle energy systems of the astral body. The astral body is a subtle energy body that surrounds the physical body and has a direct effect on it. The subtle energy systems will be outlined in detail in the next chapter.

Although Yoga was originally intended to bring you to self-realization, other by-products of its regular practice include greater mental equanimity, emotional stability and physical rejuvenation.

In addition it also increases strength and flexibility, reduces stress and tension, builds stamina and develops focus. Yoga also enables you to practice detachment. Yoga's greatest gift is that it presents you with an opportunity to become aware of the subconscious thoughts and emotions that lead to emotional, mental and physical dis-ease.

How the Spiritual Discipline of Yoga Works

Here is one explanation of how the Spiritual discipline of Yoga can help you to experience Radiant Health. Reactions can cause you to hold your breath. Holding the breath stops you from fully experiencing the sensation in each of the three bodies. At the point the breath is held, the emotional, mental or physical pain is repressed or denied. The energy then becomes lodged in some part of your cellular structure (such as muscles, tissues or organs) and stored in the subconscious mind.

Blocked energy causes emotional or mental dis-eases that can lead to injuries, accidents, illness and ossification or adhesions. By combining Asanas and Pranayamas the breath brings you into the moment, enabling you to be present to what you are feeling. Also, adhesions and ossification in muscles, tissue and organs can be relieved, as can the energy blockages in the Nadis, Meridians and Chakras. Prana can be directed into the blockages as you inhale, and loosened, dissolved or completely expelled from the physical body as you exhale.

Using Pranayama to Detect and Release
Stress and Tension

You can use Pranayama to become aware of the places in the body where you carry stress and tension. Scan the body while practicing conscious breathing. Start at the top of your head and work down through the body. Notice the neck, shoulders, arms, upper, middle and lower back, gluteals, hamstrings, calves and feet. Draw the breath into the stress or tension and release it as you exhale.

Practicing Yoga reduces stress and tension and enables the body to become stronger, more supple and flexible. Dissolving long-standing injuries, muscle adhesions or ossification might take more time. Yoga is a process. Be patient and in time you will experience more peace, acceptance and tolerance.

Your Asana Practice Is a Microcosm of Life

When you engage in a regular Asana practice, you will notice how it reflects life. There will be movements that you will like, and others that you will not. Some days you will be more flexible, strong and balanced, other days you will not. Some days everything will irritate you, and other days everything will feel good. Yoga can be very confrontive to the ego. Yoga enables you to practice being a little less reactive in challenging situations, and to be a little more compassionate and accepting of who you are and where you are in your practice. It enables you to detach from the unhealthy thoughts and emotions that arise as a result of the practice.

When your breathing becomes synchronized with your movements, you will experience a meditation in motion. The practice not only increases your physical flexibility, strength and stamina but challenges you, through the intensity of the poses, to maintain mental equanimity and emotional tranquillity.

Yoga, Exercise and The Journey to Radiant Health

The intention to create Radiant Health is more important than the type of exercise you choose. Remember that life is a journey, not a destination. Especially in relationship to exercises, there is nowhere to get to—just be present with you. You do not need to be thinner, stronger or faster to be healthy. As an integrative exercise, Yoga will harmonize the three bodies, and your competitive desires can be kept to a minimum.

The Second Layer: The Physical Body's Subtle Energy Systems

The physical body is surrounded by the astral body, a subtle energy body comprised of three distinct subtle energy systems: Nadis, Chakras and Meridians. The subtle energy systems of the astral body receive and transmit pulses of light. The light, which at a basic level is information, is then deciphered and translated into the language of sensation.

The mental and emotional bodies (which are contained within the astral body) produce thoughts and emotions, which in turn exert a subtle energetic pressure on the physical body. This pressure is experienced in the physical body as sensations. The energy that flows through your physical body is interrupted when you react to the subtle or gross sensations you experience—your own or other people's conscious or subconscious emotions or thought forms.

Reactions cause interruptions.

Interruptions result in blockages.

Blocked energy leads to dis-ease.

If you do nothing to restore the flow of energy, dis-ease will eventually manifest.

Nothing disrupts the free flow of energy in the subtle and physical bodies quicker than resisting your own heart's truth. Nothing restores the free flow of energy quicker than following your heart's truth. Follow the adage *"To thine own self be true,"* and your subtle energy systems will always flow freely.

And, the highest Truth is to put Love into every Action.

DIS-EASE

The underlying cause of dis-ease is blocked energy. Dis-ease can manifest in the emotional, mental or physical body, or in all three bodies simultaneously. However, the genesis of dis-ease follows a standard operating pattern: the mental body stifles the free flow of emotional body energy.

In other words, the mental body causes all dis-ease.

However, all dis-ease begins in the emotional body.

When the emotional and mental body, feminine and masculine energy, and heart and mind are in harmony, the mind listens to and carries out the heart's messages. When harmony exists, balance is assured and Radiant Health follows. However, when the heart speaks and fear arises, the mind's power is used to invalidate, repress or deny the heart's feelings and messages, rather than being used to support the heart and identify, acknowledge and move through the fear.

Separation of heart and mind lies at the core of all dis-ease.

On the surface, emotional body dis-eases are related to repressed anger and sadness, which materialize as the emotions on the non-centered scale in the Anger and Sadness triangles (see pages 102 and 110.) Mental body dis-eases are related to unloving thought forms and include conflict, confusion and obsessions. Physical body dis-eases are related to toxic foods and substances, and manifest in stress, tension, heart dis-ease and cancer.

However, because all three bodies are interconnected, dis-ease begun in one can produce dis-ease in all.

The effects of dis-ease will be temporary when you move expeditiously to identify and eliminate its root cause. If the root cause is not uncovered, the blocked energy can fester for months or years, until it materializes as an advanced stage of physical dis-ease. In these instances, health and well-being quickly deteriorate and are difficult to restore.

The Difference in Approach Between East and West

Oriental medicine supports the theory that the root cause of all dis-ease is blocked energy. When you experience pain, the body is sending you a message that something is out of balance. The pain can be from an injury, illness, dark thoughts or emotions, or acute, chronic or life-threatening dis-ease. The pain informs you that a blockage of energy exists somewhere within one or more of the three bodies.

You can uncover the underlying cause of the dis-ease by deciphering the codes contained in an emotional or mental disturbance, or physical injury, accident or illness. This can be accomplished by identifying the affected body parts, organs or muscles as well as the dis-ease's characteristics. How to do this will be discussed in detail in the upcoming Meridian and Chakra sections. Unravel the clues and you can take measures to restore balance.

For thousands of years masculine energy has been in a position of dominance. This imbalance is responsible for the chronic state of dis-ease affecting the collective consciousness of humanity. The Eastern healthcare systems, the most ancient systems for treating illness, are viewed as the best health systems because of their holistic focus and integrative foundations. Yet even they have been greatly affected by the dominance of masculine energy. For example, in the Meridian system information in the Appendix you will find the emotional causations for dis-ease; however, it is rare to work with an Acupuncturist that will identify or address the emotional causes for physical dis-eases. A "hands off" attitude is often taken when it comes to addressing the part that emotions—a feminine construct—play in relationship to dis-ease. However, when you treat the body, and do not address either the emotional or mental causes, then core-level healing cannot take place. Core-level healing takes place when you identify the root cause of a dis-ease and work to dissolve it.

The dominance of masculine energy also affects the Western healthcare system.

A Healthcare Industry That Only Treats Dis-ease

Western medical institutes are second to none when it comes to handling emergencies and traumas, such as setting a broken leg, tending to a gunshot wound or removing a ruptured appendix. The West has also developed drugs that can provide immediate relief from the pain incurred during these episodes.

Medication can provide relief in non-emergency cases, but it is often superficial and temporary. When the focus is placed on uncovering and eradicating the root cause of the dis-ease, it will be less likely to crop up again. However, driven by greed (masked as the need to turn a profit), the masculine-energy-dominated, multi-billion-dollar healthcare industry devotes the lion's share of its financial resources to the research and development of moneymaking drugs. Drugs can treat the superficial symptoms of illness and trauma, but do not address or facilitate core-level healing.

Typically, this translates into poor and ineffective healthcare.

The pharmaceutical industry, which also operates for profit, invents, patents and sells big moneymaking drugs, such as AZT, Viagra and Prozac. The need to produce profits leaves little room to support the research, production and promotion of natural, herbal or homeopathic remedies, because they cannot be patented and are not as profitable as drugs.

This approach does little to facilitate holistic health.

It Is Time to Promote Wellness

Radiant Health is promoted when the focus shifts from treating symptoms to identifying and eliminating the root causes of dis-ease. Even well intentioned M.D.s can fall under the pharmaceutical spell of prescribing medicines and drugs that are designed to treat symptoms, rather than studying, applying and teaching wellness techniques. To avoid falling into this trap, do not turn the responsibility for your health and well-being over to others; instead empower yourself. Be accountable for your health and well-being.

Radiant Health becomes possible when you make holistic health—emotional, mental, physical and Spiritual—a priority. Design your own program to maintain your own physical, emotional and mental health and well-being. Be an active participant in your healing process. Work side by side with your primary healthcare practitioners. Do your own research and ask probing questions.

You are your own best doctor and healer.

The conventional Western model used to treat cancer is not holistic in its scope and illustrates that the treatment of dis-ease using a non-holistic approach does little to effect healing.

A Healthcare Model Gone Astray

In 1958, Max Gerson, M.D., a pioneer in the successful use of diet therapy to cure advanced cancer, stated, *"100 years ago leukemia was unknown in the United States. Fifty years ago cancer was so seldom observed in clinics and autopsies that every case was worthy of publication."*[1]

Today, cancer is a household word.

Cancer's root causes include: air and water toxicity, chronic stress and fatigue, the repression or denial of emotions, diets high in trans-fatty acids, food additives, preservatives, herbicides and pesticides, and meat and dairy products laced with antibiotics, estrogen and other growth hormones. Rather than working aggressively to eradicate its root causes, however, the medical industry devotes most of its time, energy and money to the treatment of cancer symptoms.

Although all treatments deserve fair and equal consideration when it comes to cancer, the conventional medical protocol demonstrates a healthcare system gone astray. The primary objective of healing is to uncover the root cause of dis-ease, which includes exploring and considering all possible healing modalities and protocols—then selecting the best methodologies, substances and treatments to eradicate its roots.

In the West, this ideal has been compromised.

Driven by ego behaviors such as envy, ignorance, prejudice, arrogance, pride and greed, the primary objective of healing has been abandoned and replaced by medical politics. Information, a major contributor to the healing process, has been manipulated, suppressed and even outlawed by the medical establishment in an attempt to maintain its power, control and the status quo.

Treating Dis-ease Using a Dis-eased Model

An overwhelming amount of focus and attention is showered on the few survivors of conventional cancer treatments. For example, multiple Tour de France winner Lance Armstrong receives a significant amount of press. Ignored is the staggering amount of evidence pointing to the frighteningly destructive nature of the treatments and the deadly results that occur in the majority of cases.

Conventional medical therapy for the treatment of cancer consists of surgery (cutting), radiation (burning) and chemotherapy (poisoning). The results of this treatment protocol are destructive, demoralizing and all too often deadly.

According to science writer Peter Barry Chowka, *"We've lost the war on cancer. Since the 1950's the outlook for most cancer patients has remained the same: a one in three chance of living for five years after diagnosis using conventional therapies: surgery, radiation, chemotherapy, drugs. The fact is that today two out of three American cancer patients will be dead before five years."* [2]

Dr. Virginia Livingston-Wheeler states, *"Irradiation and chemotherapy patients often have their immune systems so disrupted that they contract infectious diseases, such as pneumonia, from which they die before the cancer has a chance to kill them."* [3]

Harold Harper, M.D., author of *How You Can Beat the Killer Diseases*, said, *"The use of radiation or poison in the effort to get at the actual malignant cells is the equivalent of turning a blow torch on a wart."* [4]

Max Gerson, M.D., stated, *"To remove the underlying cause and accomplish the cure of cancer means the re-establishment of the whole metabolism, especially of the liver."* [5]

The presence of cancer is an indicator that the liver is in poor working order. A healthy and fully functioning liver is essential for clearing toxins from the blood. The toxic effects of radiation and chemotherapy seriously impair an already poorly functioning liver, often exacerbating liver function to the extent that the treatment is responsible for the liver's failure. The liver can be detoxified and restored to full health. The Liver Meridian section in the Appendix contains a number of holistic methods.

Also, a strong, healthy and fully functioning immune system is essential for the cancer fight. Surgery strains and weakens the immune system while radiation and chemotherapy wipe it out. To overcome cancer, the eliminatory organs and immune system must be strengthened so that they can attack the cancer and eliminate toxins from the body. The Appendix contains nine immune boosting nutrients that can help ward off malignant invaders. Many M.D.s are now declaring: surgery, radiation and chemotherapy are not the best weapons for the battle.

Successful Cancer Treatments Outlawed

Even more alarming are the political government authorities and entities such as the American Medical Association (AMA) and Food and Drug Administration (FDA) that reject, ban or outlaw successful, effective and natural cancer treatments and therapies without so much as an investigation.

"The Fitzgerald Report," given to Congress in the 1950s, named at least a dozen promising treatments that were blocked by organized medicine. The congressional committee came to the conclusion that a conspiracy was being perpetrated by organized medicine to suppress immunological or nutritional cancer therapies.

Consider the story of Harry M. Hoxsey, who was named in the report. In 1924, Hoxsey, a former coal miner with an eighth grade education, opened his first cancer clinic. Hoxsey used a cancer curing herbal formula developed by his great-grandfather and handed down to him by his father. The formula contained herbs used by Native Americans to cure cancer. Every species of plant used in Hoxsey's formula was covered in Jonathan Hartwell's *Plants Used Against Cancer.*[6] Hartwell was a chemist employed by the National Cancer Institute.

By the 1950s Hoxsey had centers in 17 states and his center in Dallas, Texas, was the largest privately-owned cancer treatment center in the world. Hoxsey's treatment cured tens of thousands of people. Hoxsey's centers drew over 300 people a day for treatment. Those who investigated him and those he cured, including senators, judges and even some doctors, endorsed Hoxsey's treatment.

Hoxsey's reward for curing cancer: he was labeled a quack.

By the end of 1924 Hoxsey had been arrested more times than anyone in medical history. A Dallas prosecutor, assistant district attorney Al Templeton, personally arrested Hoxsey over 100 times during a two-year period. Ironically, Templeton later became a leading proponent of the Hoxsey treatment, as well as Hoxsey's lawyer, after his brother Mike was cured by Hoxsey's treatment.

Two Federal Courts Reach the Same Conclusion: The Hoxsey Treatment Cures Cancers

Dr. Morris Fishbein, head of the *Journal of the AMA*, led the persecution of Hoxsey. Fishbein, the AMA and the FDA were responsible for an ongoing campaign of smear tactics against Hoxsey. When Fishbein, the AMA and Hearst publications called Hoxsey *"a ghoul feasting on the flesh of the dead and dying"* and *"the greatest quack of the twentieth century,"* Hoxsey brought a libel and slander suit against them.

Prior to the lawsuit, Hoxsey had formally tested his treatment on cancer patient and police sergeant Tomas Mannings in front of Fishbein and AMA officials. During the trial, Fishbein and the AMA were forced to admit that Hoxsey's external paste cured cancer. After exhaustive testimony, two federal courts concluded that Hoxsey's treatment did indeed cure cancer.

For years, Hoxsey pleaded with the medical establishment to conduct a formal scientific investigation of his treatment. Yet even after Hoxsey won two federal cases, the National Cancer Institute still refused to perform a scientific investigation on his formula. With people flocking to the Hoxsey clinics in unprecedented numbers to seek cancer treatment, the government took unprecedented action.

All 17 Hoxsey clinics were shut down, outlawed by the FDA.

The one remaining clinic now operates in Tijuana, Mexico.

Today, the only way to find out about the Hoxsey clinic is by word of mouth. Throughout its history, the Hoxsey clinic has maintained an amazing cure rate of 80%. Sadly, the cure rate is unverifiable by the medical establishment because its authorities continue to refuse to investigate the treatment.

Healing Dis-ease

In the Hoxsey treatment, the herbal paste was only the first step. Attitudinal healing and diet therapy was also used to complete the holistic treatment protocol. The eradication of dis-ease requires addressing each of the three bodies. Healing starts in the emotional body by changing dis-ease-producing belief systems, emotions and attitudes. Healing continues in the mental body, by replacing diseased thought forms with prayer, mantras and positive affirmations. In the physical body, eating habits are changed. If medicine has to be taken, be sure to supplement it with foods and herbs that support and enhance liver, kidney, eliminatory and immune system function.

Change Your View of Dis-ease

Rather than view dis-ease as an inconvenience or punishment, consider it a teacher. Illness, injury or any other form of dis-ease presents you with an opportunity to slow down, take stock of yourself, examine your situation and reestablish your natural rhythm and cycle. For example, you can use the illness to uncover and transform the thoughts, emotions, beliefs or behaviors that led to it. Take the common cold for example. Generally, those who believe in a *"cold and flu season"* get ill during that period. Those who do not subscribe to the belief system stay healthy. If you catch a cold, examine your thoughts and beliefs and know that you have the power to change.

Another way to support your health and well-being or relieve dis-ease is to keep the subtle energy in the Nadis, Meridians and Chakras flowing freely.

NADIS, MERIDIANS AND CHAKRAS

The discovery that the physical body is comprised entirely of light is a relatively recent breakthrough in the scientific field of quantum physics.

But Yogis and Sages have known this for thousands of years.

Using meditation as their primary method of investigation, Yogis detected two subtle energy bodies, in addition to the physical body. Yogis discovered that the astral body enveloped physical body, and that the astral body was encased in the causal body. The astral body contains the emotional and mental bodies, as well as three subtle energy systems. The three subtle energy systems include:

The Nadis: *72,000 individual energy points.*

The Meridians: *12 internal and external energy pathways.*

The Chakras: *7 spinning vortex disks of energy.*

Yogis experimented on the body to validate their findings. When the accuracy of their findings was confirmed, healing systems based on the original blueprints were developed and put into use. Today, the original subtle energy systems' blueprints serve as the foundations of what are, arguably, the oldest healing systems in the world: Ayervedic and Acupuncture.

The Nadi, Meridian and Chakra systems are the subtle energy systems that maintain the integrity of the three bodies. In the upcoming sections, you will learn the basics about each of these three systems. In the Appendix, you will find complete and detailed information regarding the Meridian and Chakra systems. You will also learn meditation techniques to alleviate blockages from these energy systems.

The power of meditation is key to keep these subtle energy systems open and flowing freely. By using meditation to turn your attention inward, you can learn to recognize and expose the roots of dis-ease before they manifest in illness. You can then take action to eliminate the blockages before they grow into full-fledged dis-ease.

NADIS

The Nadis are a subtle energy system that consists of 72,000 stationary points. Contained in the astral body, the Nadis are an integrated matrix of individual points that receive and transmit pulses of light. The Nadis are like subtle veins and arteries. The pulses of light received by the Nadis are translated into information and then sent to the Chakras where they can be deciphered by the truth centers: instinct, intuition and heart. Each Nadi governs specific emotional, mental and physical functions, but practically speaking, the Nadis are too numerous to discuss individually. To study each point and its specific meaning and effects would be an overwhelming task.

To satisfy the purpose of understanding the subtle energy systems of the astral body and their functions, the Meridian and Chakra systems will provide a more than adequate amount of information.

MERIDIANS

The Meridians comprise twelve distinct energy pathways that traverse the internal and external physical body. Each Meridian rules a specific internal organ—which is either Yin or Yang in nature. The six Meridian pairs also govern specific emotional and mental patterns and physical body functions. Acupuncture and Acupressure use the Meridians to balance the subtle energy bodies of patients, thereby facilitating healing.

After an illness or injury has been identified, and its location on or inside the body pinpointed, the dis-ease can be traced to its corresponding Meridian. When the Meridian that governs the dis-ease has been identified, the emotional or mental root of the dis-ease can be uncovered. At that point, proactive steps can be taken to remedy the root cause of dis-ease. These steps include eliminating negative thought patterns, expressing denied or repressed emotions and/or removing unhealthy substances from your diet. When the energy flow is restored, holistic health and well-being will return.

The Six Meridian Pairs

The meridians express nature's duality. They are partnered in six corresponding pairs according to the principles of Yin and Yang and each Meridian has an internal and external pathway. A complete overview of each of the twelve Meridians, including a separate chart for each Meridian, can be found in the Appendix, which begins on page 323. The Meridian pairs—Yin first, then Yang—are listed below. The Meridian charts are outlined in the same order as is found here:

1. Lung and Large Intestine   2. Spleen and Stomach
3. Heart and Small Intestine   4. Kidney and Bladder
5. Pericardium and Triple Warmer 6. Liver and Gall Bladder

The Appendix presents information about how to use foods, thoughts, emotions, herbs, colors, gems and crystals to keep each Meridian's energetic pathways open and performing at their peak.

CHAKRAS

The Sanskrit word *Chakra* means "wheel" or "disk." The seven Chakras compose another astral body subtle energy system. Each Chakra regulates a number of specific physical functions, as well as emotions and thought forms. The Chakras open and close to varying degrees in direct relation to your internal and external environment including healthy or dis-eased thought forms, emotions or physical states of being.

The Chakras act as intersections for the Nadis. Chakras also spin in a clockwise direction. Feelings, thoughts and actions that arise from the heart keep the Chakras' energy clear and sharp. If the rotation of the Chakras is tight and their energy pure, you will experience physical well-being, mental clarity and emotional stability. When the Chakras spin slowly and leak energy, imbalance occurs leading to physical, mental or emotional dis-ease.

Meditation Can Clear Negative Energy from the Chakras

As pure light energy, each Chakra emits a unique frequency that translates into a specific color. Because the spectrum of color emitted by light carries a very high frequency, you can raise your frequency and dissolve energy blockages by meditating on any Chakra and its ruling color.

When meditating on a Chakra, redirect its rotation and visualize it spinning in a counter-clockwise direction to clear negative or stagnant energy. When the Chakra has been cleared, its color will appear brighter and you will feel lighter. Reverse the Chakra's rotation and visualize it spinning in a clockwise rotation. This locks in its brightness and free-flowing energy, and restores its proper rotation direction. Meditating on the Chakras assists the healing process and reestablishes the free flow of your emotional body's creative energy.

A complete description of the colors of light and their meanings can be found in the Appendix. Also in the Appendix, you will find three distinct Chakra configurations: the traditional Yang/masculine Chakra system, the Yin/feminine Chakra system and the Divine Child Chakra system. Clearly illustrated and detailed, each Chakra system contains specific information on its application and the color significance associated with it. The Appendix also includes meditation practices to clear stagnant or negative energy, raise your vibration and integrate the three bodies.

Epilogue to the Nadis, Meridians and Chakras

When you feel the initial pangs of physical discomfort or oncoming illness, observe the body parts or areas being affected. Find the affected body part or location—such as nose, arm, stomach, throat, lungs or back—in the Index. Then, go to that section in the Appendix to find information on the restorative effects of gems, crystals and colors; the life-force enhancing properties of tonic herbs; and a number of meditations that are appropriate to the restoration of subtle energy system flow.

If you identify the root cause of the dis-ease as being a mental or emotional conflict, put the Meridian chart's mental and emotional harmonizers into practice. Also, use a combination of the other healing elements specific to the issue. For example, meditate using the colors and Chakra configurations specific to the emotional or mental issue. Also, wear or meditate with crystals or gems, drink tonic herbal teas, or massage the associated Meridian energy lines or body areas.

An ancient Chinese proverb states, *The wise doctor treats his patients before illness occurs.* Like a wise doctor, you can learn to look beneath the surface, listen carefully and decipher the body's subtle electro-magnetic energy pulses. The body is an instrument filled with the kind of information that can increase your awareness and help you recognize and dissolve energy blockages before they manifest into dangerous dis-eases.

Scan the body during meditation and learn to recognize signals such as tiredness, hunger, restlessness, anger, sadness or frustration. These indicate your subtle energy flows are not in harmony. When you recognize an imbalance, take an appropriate action. Rest, eat, exercise, change your thoughts and information sources, strengthen your Will, heal unhealthy emotions and experiences or redirect your Passion to restore harmony.

Work on the subtle energy systems, and a dis-ease will likely begin to dissipate or be relieved altogether. However, this information should not be used as a substitute for proper medical treatment. These methods also can be used in conjunction with professional treatment. Awareness is the key. A list of Healing Arts Professionals can be found on page 317.

33

The Physical Body Center: Action and Service

The seventh step on *The Journey to Radiant Health* is to serve, and each new day presents you with opportunities to do that when you put love into action. Put love into action and you will have a profound impact on everyone, including people you might never meet.

This is the essence of the seventh step.

Service is a powerful way to put love into action. History is filled with stories of ordinary and extraordinary individuals whose impact on the world is timeless. Their commitment to service propelled them beyond seemingly insurmountable obstacles, and their actions displayed courage and vision. They surrendered their desires and, in some instances, even sacrificed their own lives to make a difference in the lives of those they served. The list below contains some powerful and inspirational, albeit sometimes controversial, examples of what happens when people follow life's highest purpose: to serve. The point is that each person, in his or her own way, put love into action.

Mother Teresa, Malcolm X, Joan of Arc, Martin Luther King Jr., Harriet Tubman, Chief Seattle, Susan B. Anthony, Cesar Chavez, Nelson Mandela, Rosa Parks, William Wallace, Gloria Steinem, Gandhi, Geronimo, Bobby Seale and Huey P. Newton are a few examples of the countless number of individuals who chose to pursue an exalted vision of service.

The pursuit of their vision inspired countless lives and uplifted their community. Each individual made a clear, deliberate and conscious choice to shine a beacon of light on the human condition and work to achieve a higher standard for all. They challenged themselves, and every one who knew them, to live from the heart and lead a deliberate life of action and service, founded on compassion and courage, discipline and integrity, faith and trust, and love and truth.

Whether your life's purpose brings you notoriety is not as important as realizing that your life's purpose is just as significant and meaningful.

Your actions do matter.

Your General Life's Purpose

Every human being who incarnates on the planet comes to carry out a life purpose that, in essence, can be divided into two sub-purposes. The first is a broad sweeping purpose that involves all your interactions and can be displayed in all relationships.

The first sub-purpose is known as your *general life's purpose.*

Your general life's purpose is to love every sentient being on the planet. This means being respectful and considerate, showing reverence and honoring that everyone and everything you come into contact with on your journey is a part of God. Your daily activities provide ample opportunities to fulfill your general life's purpose.

Before taking any action, take the time to identify any thoughts or emotions that arise from fear that can keep you from modeling love. Use prayer to ascertain the answer to this question: *"Will the action I am about to take exemplify Agape and serve the highest good of all involved?"* Draw your focus into the heart and ask the question over and over until the mind is saturated. Next, sit quietly in meditation, dive into the stillness of your heart and patiently wait for Spirit to reveal the answer.

An action arising from the heart is always founded in love.

An action born of the ego is always founded in fear.

Some of the most potent and effective displays of loving actions come through basic and simple gestures. Listed below are seven simple and yet profound actions that can be put into action on a daily basis to express love and bring more peace and harmony into your life and the lives of others.

SEVEN ACTIONS TO PROMOTE PEACE AND HARMONY

1. *Start with a Warm Greeting.*

When meeting a family member, friend, associate or stranger, start with a warm greeting. If you use a handshake, make it firm and friendly.

A warm greeting shows genuine interest and a sincere desire to make contact. When you greet with a phrase like *"Good to see you"* or *"How are you?"* and add *"Do you need anything?"* or *"How can I help you?"* it shows that you care. Simple physical contact such as a handshake or a touch to the shoulder is a way to help others feel included and is another way to transmit your heart's love into your greeting.

2. *Smile As Often As Possible.*

A genuine smile is naturally uplifting, and transmits love, warmth and comfort. Smiling also is important to your overall well-being because its biochemical reaction stimulates neurotransmitters in the brain that promote the release of endorphins and peptides that can shift your emotional state.

The exalted Indian sage Paramahansa Yogananda said, *"If you feel that you can't smile, stand before a mirror and with your fingers pull your mouth into a smile. It's that important."*[1] In research done at the University of California at San Francisco, manic-depressive patients took part in a study to determine whether smiling could help alleviate depression. After being asked to maintain a smile for twenty minutes during a one-hour session, 80% of the patients experienced feelings of exhilaration. After practicing the routine on a daily basis for two weeks, many of the patients overcame their condition.

3. *Give Hugs As Often As You Can.*

A hug is a deeper and more intimate form of physical contact. Hugs can convey feelings of warmth and a sense of safety and security. A hug can help you feel calm and relaxed during a stressful time or in a tense environment. A hug also can convey your excitement, joy and happiness.

Although everyone can benefit from the physically nurturing contact of a hug, this level of intimate contact can be uncomfortable or overwhelming for some people. If you want to give someone a hug and are not sure if it's okay, ask first. This provides others the safety and freedom to say *"yes"* or *"no."* Here are some rules of thumb when giving or receiving hugs:

1. *Do not pat the back when giving a hug. Giving a hug is not akin to burping a baby!*

2. *A hug should be firm, not overbearing or forceful.*

3. *Breathe fully during a hug to take in the love, warmth, comfort and reassurance it conveys.*

4. *Hug until your hearts find the same beat.*

5. *Do not hug out of obligation.*

6. *In every hug there is a natural release point; when you feel it, let go.*

7. *If you want or need a hug, ask for one!*

4. *Make Eye Contact.*

The eyes are the windows to the Soul. Making eye contact conveys confidence, interest, caring and sincerity. It lets others know that you are paying attention. Soft gazes project love, while penetrating looks and staring can be intimidating. Also, be sure to take off your sunglasses when talking to someone; let them see the love in your heart as it shines through your eyes.

When you are dealing with an angry person, avoid direct eye contact but do not look away. Soften your gaze and drop your eyes to their throat or heart level. In this way the vibration of their anger will not affect you. You allow them the space and safety to vent, knowing that they have your full and undivided attention, while you maintain the integrity of your own higher, loving vibration.

5. *Listen with an Open Heart and Mind.*

Effective listening is truly an art. It actually can appear to be a passive behavior, but it is one of the most powerful of all loving actions. Listening is a nurturing and healing action that lets others know that you care.

People often need to talk to vent their feelings or resolve their confusion. Listen with an open heart and you will move beyond the spoken words. Openhearted listening enables you to access the more sensitive, intuitive and empathic place within you. Listen with the heart and you will gain greater insight and a deeper and more complete understanding of what is really being said and what the speaker really needs. Give your complete and undivided attention and others will know that you are sincere and engaged in the moment.

Native Americans say that we have two ears and one mouth as a reminder to listen twice as much as we speak. Take the time to listen and you can provide a true and essential balm to ease the pain and suffering of others.

6. *Speak in Positive Terms.*

It is often easy to express the negative rather than accentuate the positive. This is especially true when your feelings have been hurt or you have been treated with disrespect. This does not mean to deny the truth of a situation. Nonetheless, if you cannot say something positive, then do the next best thing—remain silent.

Silence enables you to internalize your focus and reestablish contact with your heart. Being silent also can stop you from engaging in gossip. Because we are empathic, kinetic and telepathic beings, gossip emits a lower vibration that is harmful to both the gossiper and the gossipee.

The more positive words you can speak, the higher the overall vibrations you will put into the ethers. As a result, you will reap the positive feelings those vibrations create. Speaking in positive terms also can help uplift others and help them to find the good in a situation, even when it might appear negative.

7. *Maintain a Reverent Attitude.*

A reverent attitude is a display of genuine humility. Reverence reminds us that everyone and everything in the world is important, and is a container of God Itself. A reverent approach honors that everyone has a place of significance in God's universe.

Reverence reminds you to look for the reflection of God in every human being. A reverent attitude creates the kind of safe, stable and nurturing environment that makes it possible for you to serve others. A reverent attitude enables you to drop the ego and express the authentic and genuine wonder and awe for all of God's creations.

Your Life's Specific Purpose

While the first part of your life's purpose is broad, sweeping and involves all your interactions and relationships, the second part is more precise and defines the scope of your own personal and Spiritual growth opportunities.

The second part of your life's purpose is known as your *specific life's purpose.*

Your specific life's purpose has nothing to do with attaining fame or fortune, although it might bring those things to you. Instead, your specific life's purpose relates to the pursuit of a task that you will perform in service to others. Your specific life's purpose provides the reason for your incarnation on the planet and contains the primary talents or gifts that you brought to share with the world.

It is by your effort to uncover and carry out your specific life's purpose that your success can be measured. *Do what you love and the money will follow* is a popular adage. However, when you are in alignment with your life's purpose and are taking actions devoted to carrying it out, money will not be an issue. When you do what you love, Spirit will always provide for you, you always have what you need, and you will find deep satisfaction as your talents serve the needs of others.

Your specific life's purpose can be found in the Passion exercise Part I, and "The Spirit Child Contains Your Dreams."

Your specific life's purpose will challenge you in many ways to grow. The ego and its fear is the only element that can stop you from identifying, validating and carrying it out. If the ego's fear arises, reread Chapters 24 to 27. Do not let the ego win! Overcome it by reconnecting to your heart and putting Love into Action. The pursuit of your specific life's purpose can bring you a tremendous sense of fulfillment and satisfaction, as well as a great sense of achievement and freedom.

Your specific life's purpose might be to raise a son or daughter, be a counselor or be the president of a large corporation. It might be to write children's books, be a banker or be a molecular biologist. Whatever your specific life's purpose, it will never be at odds with your general life's purpose. In fact, the two support one another.

Merging Your General and Specific Life's Purpose

Combine your specific life's purpose with your general life's purpose and you will bring more positive effects to the world. Regardless of your specific life's purpose, you can use your general life's purpose to love others as well as yourself. By merging the general and specific life purpose, you can express the totality of God's love as you share it with each person you contact through your specific life's purpose.

In fact, the two can never be separate.

Doing one helps complete the other and vice versa. Joined together in a cohesive framework, your general and specific life's purposes will always give rise to feelings of peace, joy, happiness and an overall sense of well-being. Put your general and specific life's purpose into action and you can become more forgiving, accepting, compassionate and trusting towards others, yourself and life in general.

Ascertain Your Specific Life's Purpose

Your specific life's purpose might challenge you emotionally, mentally or physically, but it will not cause you misery or suffering. Your specific life's purpose often challenges you to face and overcome barriers and fears, but also fills you with a sense of accomplishment, self-respect and a greater feeling of self-worth.

If you are constantly unhappy, empty or unsatisfied in your life and/or career, it is likely that you either have not uncovered your specific life's purpose or have not made a clear commitment to carry it out. You might be doing something that is safe and comfortable. But when you look into your heart, you will know that what you are doing is not the thing that will bring you fulfillment or sustain your happiness.

If this is the case, or even if it is not, use the exercise below to help you discover what makes you happy. Life is filled with pain, but when you achieve balance, pain is put into perspective. If you have trouble finding your specific life's purpose or carrying it out, then do not hesitate to get in touch with a healing arts professional to assist you on the journey. Your health, happiness and well-being depend on it!

EXERCISE:
FINDING YOUR SPECIFIC LIFE'S PURPOSE

1. Take out the list containing your heart's Passions from Chapter 15 and your Spirit Child's dreams from Chapter 17. Somewhere in these two lists, you will find your specific life's purpose.

2. If you have not completed the lists, do so now. Do not limit yourself. Include everything you enjoy, such as bike riding, singing, painting, laughing, dancing, writing, talking to adults or kids, listening to music, fixing things, climbing trees, playing at the beach, riding horses, making up games or playing with animals.

3. Align your Will with the Divine Will—See Chapter 23

4. Ask your Spirit Child to reveal your specific purpose. Then meditate to receive the answer.

If you have trouble identifying your purpose, pray to have the fear revealed that is stopping you from recognizing it. When your specific life's purpose becomes clear, you might feel excitement, anxiety or other emotions. Embrace them all with an open heart.

5. After ascertaining your specific life's purpose, use the mental body's constructive components to help you create a plan of action.

   For example, if your life's purpose is to treat the sick, then create a plan of action based around the purpose. Your first action might be to study your options. Do you want to go to medical school, Chiropractic college or a Healing Arts school? Create short and long term plans.

6. Use the mental body's constructive components to put your plan into action and move toward its fulfillment.

7. Use the components in the center of the emotional and mental body to overcome obstacles and any fear-based resistance that arises on the journey to fulfill your specific life's purpose.

Epilogue to Finding Your Specific Life's Purpose

Your specific life's purpose is important. Serve others and you will grow in humility and become an inspirational example of love in action. The highest good and most esteemed duty and responsibility of a human being is to serve others.

As we serve others, so we serve ourselves.

SECTION SEVEN

Be The Change
You Would Like
To See In Others
—Gandhi

34

Awakening:
The Journey to Light

Life is a challenge, meet it!
Life is a dream, realize it!
Life is a game, play it!
Life is LOVE, enjoy it!

—Sai Baba

Humanity has long looked to the heavens, waiting to be rescued and wanting to be saved from the darkness of ignorance, pain and suffering. But, rather than looking to the heavens to find a savior, it is time to awaken, to look within and bring forth the savior that lives in your own heart. It is time to reclaim your divinity, dispel the darkness and take responsibility for the condition of your life.

And you have plenty of help.

With *conscious breathing* as your foundation, *putting love into action* as your focus and *prayer and meditation* as tools that connect you to Spirit, you are well equipped to deal with whatever obstacles arise on your *Journey to Radiant Health.*

But that's not all.

The loving presence of masters like Jesus, Buddha, Mother Mary, Quan Yin, the Avatar Sri Sathya Sai Baba and many more are here to provide you with answers founded in truth. All you have to do is study and contemplate their teachings, and then reach out, through prayer and meditation, to ask them to guide your journey.

The Earth is also making a contribution. Her changing vibration field (which began with the Harmonic Convergence in 1987 and continues today) is helping to fuel an unprecedented shift in the conscious awareness of human beings the world over. Practice the *Raise my vibration* meditation (see Chapter 2) and you can attune your gross and subtle bodies to match her ever-increasing frequency. When your vibration matches hers you will access higher sources of information and experience a new level of conscious awareness.

Spiritual messengers are also fueling the awakening.

Harbingers of the Light have arrived to help you make sense of the rapid changes that are taking place. Teachers are here to help you understand the effects of the shifting energy and how to use it to create positive healthy change. The harbingers have come to impart Spiritual knowledge, promote love, support the awakening process and remind you of your Divine nature.

You might even know a harbinger or two.

The harbingers are seemingly regular people with an exalted vision. Their daily actions and lives are guided by the wisdom of higher conscious awareness and the compassion that dwells in the heart. The need for power and control does not motivate them. They simply work to help you understand the spiritual principles and practices that will bring you closer to realizing your true nature as God in human form. Their actions model integrity and promote altruism, and their message will saturate your heart and mind and give you a renewed sense of hope.

The Awakening Is Gathering Momentum

With this much help, there is no need to worry or waste time fearing for the future. Everything is in Divine order. People are awakening and the evidence is everywhere. For example, attendance at personal growth lectures and seminars is soaring. Ancient wisdom from East and West is being rediscovered and put into practice. Spiritual tours to sacred sites around the world are attracting record numbers, and ceremony and ritual are allowing people to celebrate God and affirm their connection to Spirit.

In the last part of the twentieth century, sales and distribution of

Spiritual books reached all time highs, surpassing every other book category.[1] Seventy-five percent of insured individuals are choosing alternative healthcare over conventional healthcare and are willing to pay cash for it.[2] Insurance companies such as Blue Shield and Blue Cross of California now cover integrative holistic healthcare practices such as Acupuncture, Massage Therapy, Yoga and Bodywork.

As the movement towards conscious awareness gathers momentum, more and more individuals are being drawn to the light. The awakening movement is growing exponentially and eventually its momentum will reach the peak energy state described as *critical mass.* When the energy reaches *critical mass,* the collective human consciousness will undergo a spontaneous and instantaneous paradigm shift.

In that very moment a New Age will be born.

All you have to do is make a decision to participate. The work is not always easy. Anything that is out of alignment with your inherent divinity (fears and ego behaviors) will rise to the surface. But with diligence, perseverance, honesty and humility you will be able to examine and release that which does not align with the greater plan. It is in taking action that you will experience change, find peace and have a positive effect on your family, community and world.

The Hundredth Monkey Phenomenon: Critical Mass Is the Link to a Paradigm Shift

From 1952 to 1958, Ken Keyes Jr. authored a scientific social study to substantiate the postulate of *critical mass.* The study is popularly known as the *"The Hundredth Monkey Phenomenon."*

Conducted on the Japanese Macaca fuscata monkeys on the island of Koshima, the study began with scientists observing the monkeys in the wild. The scientists provided the monkeys with sweet potatoes dropped in the sand. The problem the monkeys encountered was how to remove the sand from the sweet potatoes. Eventually, an 18-month-old monkey named Imo solved the problem. She began to wash her sweet potatoes in a stream. Afterwards, she taught her mother and the other young monkeys to wash their sweet potatoes.

Reflecting the law of *free will*, some adults chose to imitate the behavior of their offspring by adapting the potato washing routine. The remaining adults continued to eat the sand-covered potatoes.

Then in the autumn of 1958, something remarkable occurred.

One more monkey was added to the number of Koshima island monkeys who already washed their sweet potatoes. Because the exact number was unknown, 99 is the number used to represent the monkeys that were already washing their sweet potatoes. When the hundredth monkey learned to wash her sweet potatoes, *critical mass* was reached. In that moment, a sudden and dramatic shift took place and by that night, nearly every monkey on the island began washing his or her sweet potatoes.

But that was only the beginning.

A Universal Shift in Conscious Awareness

Scientists on other islands, and on the mainland at Takasakiyama, reported that the Macaca fuscata monkeys suddenly began to wash their potatoes without any outside prompting or influence. As the awareness of how to wash sweet potatoes reached *critical mass,* a complete shift took place in the Macaca fuscata's collective consciousness. The shift allowed information to be transmitted directly from mind to mind, and even over the sea.

Many of the prophetic events set out in Chapter 2 have come to pass. Still others have yet to unfold. But one thing is certain: Hopi, Mayan, Lakota, Bible and Shuuka Naadi prophecies herald an approaching era that will hail peace and harmony. Many of the cornerstones are in place. Only one prerequisite remains to be carried out before the New Age unfolds. The last piece of the puzzle is a dynamic paradigm shift in humanity's collective consciousness.

Do Your Part to Facilitate the Shift

If you are reading this book then you have already made a conscious choice to focus on love and its frequency. This means that a restructuring sequence has been set in motion, and your psyche and physical and subtle energy bodies will undergo a complete repatterning. Every cell in your body—right down to your DNA—will undergo a shift in vibration, and as a result you will experience a shift in consciousness. As the vibration of Love works its way through your entire cellular structure, your old thoughts, beliefs, behaviors and actions will change.

As your vibratory rate rises, the light will expose and dislodge the dense energies, ego and fears. Face the fears straight on. Acknowledge that you are Divinity Itself, do not let the ego win and you will walk in the light of Love and the veil of darkness will lift. With the light to aid you it will be easier to contact your Guides and access higher conscious information. When fears rise to the surface, the vibration of Love will enable you to overcome them. When the ego and its illusions challenge you, the light of Love that resides in your heart and Spirit will dispel the darkness. The light of Love will also enable you to take refuge in the knowledge that all things are in Divine order.

As you begin to put Love into action, you might experience relapses in which you revert to old habits or unhealthy behaviors; but do not fret, adhere to your commitment and in time they will fade away. Prayers and mantras will keep you focused on God. Meditation will hasten the restructuring time frame, expand your conscious awareness and enable you to embody loving practices such as self-forgiveness.

To further the shift, examine your actions. Are you practicing conscious breathing and making an effort to express and embody Love? Be persistent and remember: effort, not perfection, is key.

The Dawning of a New Age

As the age of darkness comes to a close you have a decision to make. Bliss is your nature and Love is God's Will for you, but you have to decide to walk the path of Love. No one can make the decision for you, or force you to do it. Change your mind-set, put Love into action, celebrate your life, and see God in all things and treat all with respect and dignity. This will bring the New Age one step closer to reality.

The Avatar Sathya Sai Baba coined an acronym, *WATCH,* that you can apply every day to your life. Use it to keep your focus on God. Be mindful to *WATCH* your:

Words

Actions

Thoughts

Character

Heart

The *WATCH* acronym can also be turned into a simple prayer: *"Spirit please guide my words, actions, thoughts, character and heart."* Recite this prayer with passion and you will feel Spirit's presence as it enters your words, actions, thoughts, character and heart. This prayer is one way to invoke Spirit to inspire and guide the transmission of Love through you and into any situation. But any prayer to Divine Mother or Father that is invoked with passion, devotion and love will open your own heart and bring peace.

The simplest expressions of Love have the most positive effect on your life and on the lives of others. Do what you can to be of service; dedicate some of your time and resources to others and you will reduce their pain and suffering and experience joy and satisfaction. Open your heart and pray for guidance and inspiration, and then meditate. The Creator and your Angels and Guides will inspire you to great actions.

Working with a Healing Arts Professional

The exercises and practices in *The Journey to Radiant Health* can help considerably in your quest to raise your awareness. If you find that you need a little extra help to get the most out of the exercises, then consider working with a healing arts professional. A healing arts professional can provide a safe and objective environment in which you can examine your beliefs and behaviors, and identify and overcome fears, unhealthy behaviors and imprints.

The following list contains conventional and holistic healthcare professionals. Before choosing a healthcare professional, write out what you want to accomplish. The clearer you can be, the better the guidance, direction and support you will receive.

HEALTHCARE PRACTITIONERS AND HEALING ARTS PROFESSIONALS

Chiropractors. Acupuncturists. Spiritual Counselors. Yoga Instructors. Neuro-Linguistic Programmers. Naturopaths. Color Therapists. Shamans. Acupressure Technicians. Rolfers. Massage Therapists. Homeopaths. Nutritionists. Bodyworkers. Psychics. Astrologers. Hypnotherapists. Cranial Sacral Therapists. Success Coaches. Dance Movement Therapists. Psychotherapists. Poetry Therapists. Rebirthers. Medical Doctors with a holistic orientation. Herbalists. Registered Dieticians.

Because the field continues to grow, this is not a conclusive list.

A Final Review

Nurture the Emotional Body

Open your heart. Direct your passion towards creative endeavors. Express your emotions in harmonious, healthy and productive ways. Heal your emotional wounds. Do not worry about the past and future. Access the truth centers. Meditate every day. Put love into action. Practice the qualities of Agape. Forgive, accept, be compassionate and trust. Make your relationships a priority. Cultivate an attitude of gratitude and celebrate your life.

Activate the Mental Body

Open your mind. Keep your thoughts focused on love. Contemplate before you act. Consider the sources from which you gather information. Do they promote conflict, pain and fear? Or do they promote creative solutions, love and harmony? Align your Will with the Divine Will. Pray for the wisdom to express love in all your actions.

Energize the Physical Body

Breathe fully in every moment. Take part in physical activities that make your body feel good. Rest, relax and reduce your stress. Eat to nourish all three bodies. Use vitamins, herbs, tears and laughter to keep your immune system strong and healthy. Meditate on the Chakras every day and use the Colors of Light to keep them open and free of blockages.

Now Is the Time to Act

Now it is time to put what you have learned into action. Apply the exercises set forth in *The Journey to Radiant Health* and you will be catapulted into a higher state of conscious awareness. Do not fight the ego or get caught up in its illusions. Instead, breathe, pray and meditate, and exemplify the basic and exalted Spiritual elements:

> *Love and Agape in the Emotional body.*
> *Truth and Wisdom in the Mental body.*
> *Action and Service in the Physical body.*

You live in a time unlike any other. Nothing will stop the evolutionary shift in consciousness. The cycle of darkness is coming to a close and you are being bathed in the light that is Spirit. Expect the unexpected. Awaken to your true nature and:

Follow your heart. Let it sing, dance and celebrate.
Let common sense be your guide.

Surrender your attachments and
Be moderate in your activities.

Laugh as much and as often as possible.
May you be ever joy-filled and happy.

And may we meet and
Share that joy and happiness on
The Journey to Radiant Health.

SECTION EIGHT

Appendix

HEALING SYSTEMS, HERBS AND SUBSTANCES

Each of the following healing systems, herbs and substances can be used to support your healing journey. As always, however, at the first sign of pain, illness or injury, consult a professional health-care practitioner. Afterwards, you can use any combination of the Meridian, Chakra, Colors of Light or Gems and Crystals systems. The Tonic Herbs and Immune Boosting Nutrient substances can also assist your return to health.

THE MERIDIAN CHARTS

The following section contains all twelve Meridian charts. Each chart displays the Meridian's internal and external energy pathways. Broken lines indicate the Meridian's internal pathway, solid lines indicate the external pathway, and the clearly marked dots highlight the most important Meridian points. Gently press each point, using the index finger, until a pulse is clearly detected. A pulse signifies the flow of energy through the Meridian.

Each chart includes the internal organ and other body parts and areas governed by the Meridian, and the two-hour period when the Meridian's energy is at its peak. Additional information relevant to the Meridian pair includes discord-producing emotions and thought forms and their harmonizing counterparts. Also included is a list of herbs, gems, crystals and colors that can be used to synthesize the Meridian's energy and dissolve energy blockages in each of the bodies governed by the Meridian pair. The chart page also displays the element, taste and season governed by the Meridian pair. Each chart page is followed by general and detailed information that relates to the use of foods, herbs, essential oils, colors and other actions that can help integrate the three bodies and restore balance to the Meridians and their associated physical organs.

THE LUNG AND LARGE INTESTINE MERIDIANS

Meridian peak time: Lung: 3 to 5 AM Large Intestine: 5 to 7 AM
Physical Dis-eases:

Sore throat
Skin problems
Constipation
Bronchitis
Asthma
Tonsillitis
Diarrhea
Sinus problem
Congestion
Shoulder pain
Insomnia

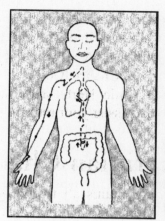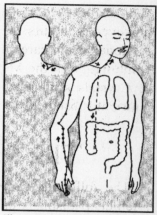

Illustrations by Christine Collings

Emotional discords:	All Sadness-related emotions Grief, Low self-esteem
Emotional harmonizers:	Compassion & Self-acceptance
Mental discords:	Toxic thoughts, Attachments
Mental harmonizers:	Letting go, Wisdom, Honor

Healing Color Associations

White (physical body)	Pink (emotional body)	Gold (mental body)

Taste: Pungent (spicy) **Element:** Metal **Season:** Autumn

Healing Gems & Crystals: Adventurine, Emerald, Garnet and Bloodstone

Herbs: American Ginseng, Astragulus, Siberian Ginseng, Codonopsis, Ginkgo Biloba, Apricot Seed, Royal Jelly, Asparagus Root, Ophiopogon

KEEPING THE LUNGS AND LARGE INTESTINE RADIANTLY HEALTHY

The Lungs

In Chinese medicine it is said that the lungs are in charge of your physical energy. And it is no wonder, when you consider that *approximately 80% of your energy comes directly from respiration.* The lungs convert air into energy. Also, oxygen is transported all the way down to the smallest parts of the lungs, the alveoli, where gases enter and leave the cells. The oxygen is transported throughout the body to be used for cell and tissue repair or cell growth. Respiration removes carbon dioxide and other gaseous waste.

The first function the body performs is an inhale breath and the last is an exhale. In Chapters 4 to 7 you learned that breath is the gateway to your experiences, but *are you aware that the average person uses only 12% of the lung's capacity?* Shallow breathing or holding the breath is a strong indicator of emotional repression or fear of losing control. Breathing deeply will cause you to feel deeply, and feelings can sometimes be difficult to handle.

Deep, free-flow breathing indicates openness and spontaneity. The emotional root cause of the lung dis-ease bronchitis is anger—at the family in general and the father specifically. Asthma's emotional root cause is feeling smothered by a parent or authority figure. Waking up during lung time, between 3 AM and 5 AM, often signifies repressed or unexpressed sadness or grief.

The essential oil from *eucalyptus* opens the lungs when rubbed on the chest. *American ginseng* is the most Yin/cool ginseng, and assists in the process of transmuting air into energy and is a great lung-strengthening tonic. However, *do not use ginseng during illness or in the presence of any lung dis-ease.*

Smooth, moist and supple skin reflects healthy lungs and large intestine.

The Large Intestine

The large intestine eliminates excess solid matter. Its walls can absorb water and have the capacity to harmonize vitamins B complex and K. Constipation can indicate a fear of letting go, or withholding emotions. Diarrhea can indicate rapid emotional processing in which the information/experiences were not properly digested.

Releasing/eliminating makes space available for new experiences. The large intestine Meridian's *Hoku-point, on the exterior side of the hand between the thumb and forefinger, can be used to release the bowels, reduce pain or eliminate headaches.* Apply a generous amount of pressure to the point for the two- to three-minute time period necessary to alleviate a headache. Place the thumb on the exterior and the forefinger on the underside of the point. Breathe deeply during the application of pressure.

Charcoal, ginger and *fennel* help reduce gas in the intestines. Charcoal is a great chelator, helping to bind toxic substances and eliminate them from the body. *Healthy intestines are associated with the three F's: Fiber, Flora and Fluids.* Fiber stimulates the large intestine, strengthens and keeps it working properly. Thriving intestinal Flora keeps infectious bacteria from attacking the system and provides the body with a small portion of its vitamin K requirement. Fluids enable nutrients to be reabsorbed into the system, allowing toxins to be flushed and keeping the intestines well lubricated.

Chlorophyll, found in all green vegetables, also keeps the intestinal tract healthy. *Ground flax seeds, apples* and *rice* are rich in fiber and can help regulate bowel movement.

For dis-eases related to the lungs or large intestine, begin conscious breathing and visualize one of these healing colors entering the Meridians: *white* for the lungs and large intestine, *pink* for sadness or grief, or *gold* for toxic thoughts or attachment issues. Meditate on the first Chakra to stimulate the large intestine, or the fourth Chakra to stimulate the lungs. Refer to page 347 for more information.

THE STOMACH AND SPLEEN MERIDIANS

Meridian peak time: **Stomach:** 7 to 9 AM   **Spleen:** 9 to 11 AM

Physical Dis-eases:

Allergies

Anorexia

Arthritis

Bloating

Bulimia

Ulcers

Insomnia

Indigestion

Muscle spasms

Blood disorders

Immune system disorders

Fatigue after exertion

Illustrations by Christine Collings

Emotional discords:	Excessive sympathy, Hopelessness
Emotional harmonizers:	Being nurtured, Asking for support
Mental discords:	Obsessions, Worry, Pensiveness, Confusion, Forgetfulness
Mental harmonizers:	Thoughtfulness, Mindfulness, Conscious breathing

Healing Color Associations:

Yellow	Lavender	Violet, Gold
(physical body)	(emotional body)	(mental body)

Taste: Sweet   **Element:** Earth   **Season:** Indian Summer

Healing Gems & Crystals: Moonstone, Amber, Carnelian, Jade, Amethyst, Ruby, Bloodstone, Jasper, Orange Citrine, Tiger Eye

Herbs: Atractylodes, Codonopsis, Poria, Ginger, Aged Citrus, Ligustrum, Astragulus, Reishi, Alisma

KEEPING THE STOMACH AND SPLEEN
RADIANTLY HEALTHY

The Stomach

The route of the stomach Meridian runs in proximity to the external sense organs: the mouth, eyes, nose, ears and skin. The stomach is associated with taking in food and nourishment. *Yin foods* such as *fruits and vegetables* are believed to lighten the body and *Yang foods* such as *meats and grains* are considered to be more grounding.

Generally speaking, eating warmer foods like soups, broths and heated foods in the winter and cooler foods like fresh fruits, salads and raw vegetables in the summer maintains the body's equilibrium. Also, eating foods natural to your geographic region benefits your health and vitality because you receive the foods' symbiotic vital energy. Drinking beverages with meals dilutes the stomach's gastric juices, slowing down the digestion process. To ensure proper digestion, do not drink beverages a minimum of 15 minutes prior to and after meals and relax after eating.

The emotional root of the dis-ease *overeating* is discontent. The emotional root of *anorexia* is anger directed at the family, marked by an overwhelming desire to disappear. The emotional root of *bulimia* is anger directed at the father. Emotional stress or worry can affect the stomach by causing indigestion, ulcers, stomachaches or bloating.

Ginger, endive, chicory and *dandelion greens* are digestive tonics. Digestive teas can be made from *ginger* or *dried orange peels*. *Chamomile, catnip, ginseng, clove, cinnamon, thyme* and *caraway* teas calm the stomach. The herbs *fennel, fenugreek, anise* and *cardamom seed* alleviate gas.

When used in a diffuser, inhalant, bath water or applied to the skin diluted with a carrier oil, essential oil from *lavender* and *sandalwood* calm the nerves. Used similarly, the essential oil from *rosemary* stimulates concentration.

The Spleen

The spleen filters old red blood cells out of the body and is the major organ of the lymphatic system. In Eastern medicine the spleen is said to be the body's central organ, influencing all five Yin organs: kidneys, heart, pericardium, liver and lungs.

The spleen is said to unify the energy received from food by way of the stomach, and air by way of the lungs; and then distribute it to the other organs. In the Western system the spleen houses the immune system, and acts to counterbalance physical or mental stress or emotional disturbance.

The spleen also is said to govern the pancreas. The pancreas releases insulin into the blood regulating the amount of sugar used in the tissues. The pancreas also controls the powerful digestive liquid sodium-bicarbonate, which it releases into the small intestine to break down proteins, fats and carbohydrates.

Warm drinks activate the spleen's energy and stimulate the appetite when you need nourishment. Beverages taken with meals slow the digestive process and can cause you to feel bloated and uncomfortable. *Excessive salads, fruits, vegetables, sugars, sweets, cold drinks, dairy products or fruit juices inhibit the spleen's ability to perform its functions*. The omega-3s found in flaxseed oil and fish can reduce spleen-related dis-eases like arthritis, tumors and high blood pressure.

Moist, hearty lips reflect a healthy stomach and spleen.

Hearty laughter, crying openly and the external use of the essential oil *bergamot* are three things that stimulate the immune system, keeping it strong and healthy. *Zinc* activates the thymus gland which is responsible for transmuting the immune system's natural killer cells into T-Cells. The thymus gland trains each T-Cell to seek out a specific antigen. *Reishi* and *astragulus,* taken together, form the most powerful herbal combination used in traditional Oriental medicine to boost the immune system. *Shitake, maitake* and *cordyceps mushrooms* also have been shown to have powerful immune system-enhancing effects.

In research conducted at the National Cancer Institute, extracts of the maitake mushroom were discovered to stop the AIDS virus from killing T-Cells. Sterols and sterolins, two of the constituents found in phytonutrients, also play a major role in controlling immune system response. Phytonutrients like sterols and sterolins keep the immune system in balance and can be found in all green vegetables. *Echinacea* is a popular immune system booster that can be used regularly, but use in accordance with the Chinese medicine adage *"Moderation in all things."* On the other hand, *Goldenseal* acts mores like an antibiotic and should not be used for more than seven to ten consecutive days because after this time period it can adversely affect the immune system.

When you feel uncomfortable, nervous, confused or worried, take a time-out. Stop whatever you are doing. Go to a quiet place, slip into a bathroom or walk outside. Close your eyes and breathe in *gold* or *violet* to soothe the mental body, *lavender* to pacify and calm the emotional body and *yellow* to relax the physical body. You can use *blue* to cool down and slow down, and *pink* to relax and open the heart.

THE HEART AND SMALL INTESTINE MERIDIANS

Meridian peak time: **Heart:** 11 AM TO 1 PM
Small Intestine: 1 TO 3 PM

Physical Dis-eases:
Chest pain
Extreme sweating
Speech disorders
Flushed face
Hypertension
Extreme thirst
Menopause
Dry cough
Heart palpitations

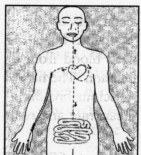 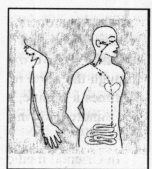

Illustrations by Christine Collings

Emotional discords: Paranoia, Melancholy
Hysteria, Acting immaturely

Emotional harmonizers: Maturity (standing in one's own power)
Being joyful, Laughter

Mental body discords: Confusion, Anxiety, Restlessness

Mental body harmonizers: Focus & Concentration

Healing color associations:

Red	Pink, Green, Magenta	Coral, Turquoise
(physical body)	(emotional body)	(mental body)

Taste: Bitter   **Element:** Fire   **Season:** Summer

Healing Gems & Crystals: Gold, Rose Quartz, Star Sapphire,
Carnelian, Red Garnet, Ruby, Orange or Brown Tourmaline,
Green Obsidian

Herbs: Reishi Mushroom (Ganoderma), Spirit Poria, Zizyphus,
Longan, Ligusticum, Pseudoginseng

KEEPING THE HEART AND SMALL INTESTINE RADIANTLY HEALTHY

The Heart

The heart continually pumps blood through the body from its four chambers. The chambers on the right side of the heart receive blood and send it to the lungs. The chambers on the left side receive oxygenated blood from the lungs and send it through the aorta for circulation. The heart beats approximately 72 times a minute, and conscious breathing can reduce its beats per minute, slowing the heart rate and reducing stress and tension.

In Oriental medicine, the *Seat of Shen*, Spirit, resides in your heart. The heart, known as the compassionate ruler, is able to see all sides of an issue. When all is well the heart is in control and you experience joy, peace and harmony. On the other hand, when your peace and tranquillity is disturbed, the heart recedes and its officials, the internal organs—containers of the impure emotions—maneuver for control.

When you feel upset or your feelings are hurt, external use of the essential oil from *patchouli* grounds your emotions. *Grapefruit* and *orange* essential oils promote cheerfulness and restore feelings of bliss and euphoria. Rub a few drops around your heart center, or put a few drops on your hands, rub them together, cup them over your nose and take some deep breaths.

In addition, you can breathe in *pink* to open your heart to unconditional love. Breathe in *green* to open your heart to truth. Use *pink* and *green* to balance the heart's feminine and masculine energies.

As your upset diminishes, breathe in the color *magenta,* which represents the highest vibrational color of unconditional love. If you find it difficult to forgive, then use the forgiveness exercises on pages 163–164. Follow it by breathing in the color *coral,* which represents the wisdom of love, and then breathe in *turquoise* to calm the mind and speak your truth from a heart infused with love.

The Small Intestine

The small intestine is in charge of the most important part of digestion, and it is divided into three portions. The upper part of the small intestine is the duodenum and it connects to the stomach. The middle part is the jejunum and the lower part, which connects to the large intestine, is the ileum. Food is partially digested by the stomach, but the majority of the digestive process occurs after it is sent to the small intestine. This is where the pancreas and gall bladder, via the liver, send digestive juices to finish the process.

The small intestine processes what it receives and sorts out the pure from the impure. The process of digestion and absorption produces energy in the form of information. The small intestine serves the heart by discarding impure thoughts and emotions and sending it the pure energy—information.

The small intestine absorbs food, salt and water into the blood. The fiber in fresh fruits, vegetables and grains helps keep the intestines functioning properly. *Fasting* gives the digestive track a rest. ***Reduce your intake of mucus-forming foods such as meats, dairy products, breads and sugars*** to keep the intestines healthy and properly prepared for digestion and assimilation.

Sweet speech, a happy face and decisions that take into account the highest good of all involved indicate a healthy heart and small intestine.

THE KIDNEY AND BLADDER MERIDIANS

Meridian peak time: **Bladder: 3 to 5 PM** **Kidney: 5 to 7 PM**
Physical Dis-eases:

Back pain
Neck pain
Sciatica
Impotence
Menstrual and
Fertility disorders
Joint pain
Knee pain
Night sweats
Chronic fatigue
Skeletal problems
Afternoon fatigue
Central nervous system and sexual disorders

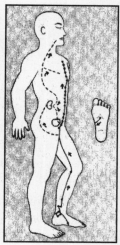

Illustrations by Christine Collings

Emotional discords:	Fear, Guilt, Shame, Hoarding
Emotional harmonizers:	Courage, Trust, Giving and Sharing
Mental discords:	Not being able to listen, Stubbornness, Rigidity
Mental harmonizers:	Introspection, Adaptability, Will, Ambition

Healing Color Associations:

Blue	Red	Red	Coral
(physical body)	(emotional body)	(mental body)	(sexual organs)

Taste: Salty   **Element:** Water   **Season:** Winter

Healing Gems & Crystals: Smoky Quartz, Copper, Bloodstone, Hematite, Emerald, Jade, Amber, Citrine

Herbs: Rehmannia, Morinda, Ho Sho Wu, Epimedium, Lycium, Schizandra, Polygonatum sibericum, Eucommia, Gecko, Dendrobium, Cnidium, Ligustrum, Astragulus, Deer antler tips

KEEPING THE KIDNEYS AND BLADDER
RADIANTLY HEALTHY

The Kidneys

The kidneys are referred to as the *"gate of life"* and are said to store your life force energy. **The kidneys filter waste and water at the rate of approximately 50 gallons of blood per hour.** Water and other useful materials are reabsorbed by the blood, and the wastes are sent to the bladder for elimination. The kidney's three main functions are to excrete waste, maintain the balance of water in the system and maintain the acid-alkaline balance.

The kidneys control the adrenals, the power and function of the brain, hair, sexual organs and skeletal system including the bone marrow which is responsible for production of white, immune blood cells. Agility, strength and a sparkle in the eyes indicate healthy kidneys. When the kidneys are weak, dark lines appear just below the eyes and you will experience lethargy or exhaustion. *Ice cold beverages or being cold adversely affect the kidneys and can produce or intensify fear or anxiety.*

Caffeine provides the kidney-ruled adrenals with a short term energy surge called a false fire. It is called a false fire because the caffeine by-passes the kidneys, firing the adrenals directly. In the long run, a false fire depletes your vital life force energy. A healthy alternative is to take a nap or do a short meditation. Teas made from *ginseng, licorice, sarsaparilla, burdock* or *comfrey* stimulate the kidney's energy. Teas made from herbs such as *morinda, lycium, rehmannia, ho sho wu* and *polygonatum sibericum* replenish the kidney's life force energy. External application and use of the essential oils from *peppermint* and *rosemary* invigorate the kidneys and combat afternoon fatigue.

During the kidney's peak period, as well as during winter, activities such as getting rest, keeping warm, being quiet and introspective should be given an even greater priority to preserve your life force energy.

The Bladder

The bladder temporarily stores and then releases waste fluids. It is stationed behind the pubic bone and as the bladder fills, it expands up into the abdomen. The bladder easily adapts to being empty or full, functioning like a diplomat who keeps things fluid and moving. The bladder governs your ability to adapt to change and remain flexible in the face of challenges.

The bladder is the longest and most Yang Meridian in the body, covering the entire length of the back of the body. It is viewed as the armor or protection of the body. It is said that if the bladder Meridian can be balanced, the whole body will return to balance.

The bladder Meridian can be used to release tension in all areas of the back. *Back pain* is also associated with feeling a lack of emotional support and being closed-minded to hearing new information.

Yoga, being holistic in nature, is a great practice to reduce back pain. *Yogic Asanas can help strengthen the back and abdominal muscles.* As Yoga combines breath with movement, it creates a meditation in motion. This helps release emotional and mental energy that cause pain.

Chiropractic treatment and the external use of the essential oil from *lavender* can reduce or alleviate back pain and tension. To reduce pain, alternate hot and cold packs every 10 minutes—but first check with your Chiropractor. *Cranberry juice* is often used to alleviate bladder infections.

The essential oil from *grapefruit* and *juniper* can help reduce the effects of water retention. *Sandalwood* is revered for its sexual restorative properties, while *geranium* can help soothe the effects of menopause and pre-menstrual syndrome.

Use the color *blue* to keep the kidney/bladder Meridian energy flowing freely. Breathe it in and visualize the blue moving straight into the kidneys. Use the color *red* to thaw out emotional fear and mental rigidity that can cause you to shrink away from challenges, constrict your creative energy and close your mind.

THE PERICARDIUM AND TRIPLE WARMER MERIDIANS

Meridian peak time: Pericardium: 7 to 9 PM

Triple Warmer 9 to 11 PM

Physical Dis-eases:

Carpal tunnel
  syndrome

Stroke

Fever

Exhaustion

Blurred vision

Stiff elbow/arm

Inability to grasp

Emotional discords: Heart pain due to relationship discord, Children's nightmares, Fear of intimacy, Embarrassment, Insanity

Emotional harmonizers: Trust, Expressing your feelings

Mental discords: Inappropriate laughter or communication, Shock, Loss of Control

Mental harmonizers: Willingness to risk re-opening the heart Honest communication

Healing Color Associations:

Pink	Royal blue	Coral, Turquoise
(physical body)	(emotional body)	(mental body)

Taste: Bitter   **Element:** Fire   **Season:** Summer

Healing Gems & Crystals: Moonstone, Turquoise, Fire Opal, Amethyst, Tourmaline.

Herbs: Waterfall Accorus, Asparagus Root, Polygala, Albizzia.

KEEPING THE PERICARDIUM
AND TRIPLE WARMER RADIANTLY HEALTHY

The Pericardium

The pericardium is the soft tissue sac that surrounds the heart and provides lubrication so the heart can move freely. The pericardium regulates blood flow, heat and nourishment, and protects the heart by absorbing initial traumas directed at the heart. The pericardium Meridian can be used to ease and heal trauma to the psyche in relationship to sexual dysfunction. It also brings balance to the heart and mind in sexual relationships.

When the pericardium is weakened, dis-ease can invade and affect the heart. Although each Meridian governs a number of emotional and mental dis-eases, the pericardium Meridian is the root container for all emotional/mental dis-eases.

The pericardium is described as the sergeant at arms to the royal court, the heart, because when your heart is upset the pericardium counterbalances the disturbance by taking the proverbial "blows."

Addictions such as overeating, drinking, smoking, sex, TV and drugs stem from experiencing overwhelming, unacknowledged and unexpressed emotional pain and suffering. Addictions are a sign that the pericardium is staggering from the amount of blows it has taken to protect the heart. Some of the blows include heartbreak, abuse and the unfulfilled desire to be loved and accepted. The pericardium enables you to survive the trauma, albeit with great damage to your self-esteem.

Although the pericardium's intentions are pure, it can be viewed as the lower-nature ego. The pericardium protects the heart by taking charge of an unhealthy situation and ordering the internal organs, the other officials, to hide emotional wounds and scars. The pericardium orders the other officials to do whatever is necessary to alleviate the heart's pain and suffering. When the lower-nature ego pericardium allows the other officials to repress or deny pain and emotions over a long period of time, the energy solidifies and can manifest as tumors or cancers.

When you allow the pericardium—the ego—to take control, you will constantly react in order to survive, rather than feel and grow. To break an addiction, come back to the heart—your higher-nature Spirit. Be willing to own, express and release your pain and trauma.

Also, take a risk and attend a twelve-step program that addresses your addiction. Some of the twelve-step programs include *Alcoholics Anonymous, Narcotics Anonymous, Over-Eaters Anonymous, Sex and Love Addicts Anonymous* and *Gamblers Anonymous*. Because twelve-step programs are anonymous and confidential, they provide a safe space from which you can share your experiences and be honest in your communications. Twelve-step programs enable you to create a Spiritual foundation and a heart-based support system for your recovery.

In time, you will come to trust yourself, God and others.

When the pain has been released, you can move forward and meet life with an open heart. Your creative energy flow will be restored and you will be fully prepared to experience life as it is.

By putting the pericardium's emotional and mental harmoniz-ers into action—willingness to re-open your heart, communicate honestly and express how you feel—the heart will regain its strength and power.

When you experience pain due to a relationship, express your feelings. Make teas from the herbs *asparagus root, polygala, water-fall accorus* and *albizzia*. Use the color *pink* in meditation to soothe the pain in your physical heart. Use *royal blue* in your meditation to soothe the emotional body. Use *coral* and *turquoise* in your medita-tion to soothe the mental body. Also, use as many of the substances from the heart Meridian as you can to heal your heart.

The Triple Warmer

The triple warmer regulates the energy in the three burning spaces in the body's trunk. The lungs and heart, which are the respiratory organs, are contained in the upper burner. The stomach, spleen, liver and gall bladder—which are digestive and assimilative organs—are contained in the middle burner. The kidneys, bladder and sexual organs—which are the eliminative organs—are contained in the lower burner.

The triple warmer regulates the *hypothalamus gland, appetite, endocrine system, autonomic nervous system* and *basic human drives.* It coordinates many bodily functions and also relates to the dynamics of social and family relationships.

The triple warmer also is associated with the psychic channels, especially intuition. When an emotional issue arises around your relationships and you want to get a Spiritual perspective, breathe in the color *royal blue,* focus on the sixth Chakra and ask for the highest good to be revealed.

The color *coral* represents the wisdom found in love and can be used to regain control or to stop inappropriate laughter. Follow it by breathing in the color *turquoise* to calm the mind and speak your truth from the heart.

When you feel upset or your feelings are hurt, the essential oil *patchouli* grounds your emotions, and *grapefruit* and *orange* promote cheerfulness and restore feelings of bliss and euphoria. Take a few drops and rub it around your heart center. For sensitive skin, put a few drops on a damp cloth and do the same. Or, put a few drops on your hands, rub them together, cup your hands over your nose and take a few deep breaths.

After applying the essential oils, sit quietly, focus your mind on conscious breathing and focus on opening your heart.

THE LIVER AND GALL BLADDER MERIDIANS

Meridian peak time: Gall Bladder: II PM to I AM **Liver:** I to 3 AM

Physical Dis-eases:

Eye disorders
Allergies, TMJ
Cracked nails
Migraines
Muscle spasms
Hypoglycemia
Arthritis
Ankles
Blood
Teeth grinding
Pre-menstrual syndrome

Illustrations by Christine Collings

Emotional discords: Anger-based emotions including depression

Emotional harmonizers: Being assertive, Confident, Motivated, Determined, Enthusiastic

Mental discords: Indecision, Judgment, Addictions, Compulsions

Mental harmonizers: Being creative, flexible and prepared, Making decisions

Healing Color Associations:

Green	Turquoise	Gold
(physical body)	(emotional body)	(mental body)

Taste: Sour **Element:** Wood **Season:** Spring

Healing Gems & Crystals: Emerald, Turquoise, Rose Quartz, Gold Topaz, Citrine, Lepidolite, Blue Coral, Green Obsidian

Gems & Crystals to Heal the Blood: Silver, Amethyst, Quartz

Herbs: Reishi Mushroom, Licorice, Schizandra, Royal Jelly

Herbs for the Blood: Tang Kuei, Ligusticum, Rehmannia, Peony, Longan, Red Date Jujube

KEEPING THE LIVER AND GALL BLADDER
RADIANTLY HEALTHY

The Liver

The liver is the largest organ of the body and has four lobes, the largest of which is on the right side of the body. The liver detoxifies harmful substances from the blood, breaks down fats and stores glycogen, vitamins A and D, and some of the B vitamins. The liver also forms antibodies and produces heparin, which prevents the blood from clotting.

In traditional Chinese medicine, women are said to be ruled by blood. The liver stores blood Chi (energy) and can store up to one-fourth of the body's blood supply during liver time. A woman's vitality depends on building blood and the body will not menstruate unless it has an ample supply of blood. *Eliminate cold foods, chocolate, strawberries, ice cream and sweets in general, prior to and during menstruation cycles to reduce the effects of PMS.* Regular use of *flaxseed oil* significantly reduces the chance of contracting breast cancer, and also reduces the effects of PMS. *Ground flaxseed fiber* helps to eliminate toxins.

Spicy, sour, greasy, fatty and oily foods irritate the liver. Alcohol and drugs are very harmful. Coffee stimulates the positive liver polarity of creativity, but its aromatic oils also cause central nervous system imbalances including body shakes as well as liver/gall bladder dis-eases including muscle spasms, headaches and the inability to remain calm and manage anger.

Headaches are a common side effect of coffee detoxification because the gall bladder's energy stagnates. *To eliminate coffee:* cut your consumption by half each day and take one to two capsules of *cayenne pepper.* This herb is a great blood detoxifier. Take it as needed to keep the blood energy from stagnating and prevent the headaches associated with coffee detoxification. *Codonopsis* promotes the production of blood as do herbs such as *tang kuei, ligusticum, rehmannia, peony* and *longan.*

Repressed creativity or uncontrolled anger can manifest as compulsions or addictions to alcohol, drugs, smoking, overeating, sex and gambling. The liver can be balanced by bringing your creative energy into focus and planning strategies and activities to bring more joy and love into your life.

A number of foods and herbs also can assist the liver's return to health or the improvement of its function. *Fresh carrot juice* strengthens liver function, and a quart or more a day of *beet juice* including the tops will help those who suffer from hepatitis. *Milk thistle* is one of the few substances that not only regenerates liver cells but is mild enough to be used on a daily basis. Its active constituent, Silymarin, has been shown in research to effectively prevent and reverse the harmful effects of hepatitis and cirrhosis. Because Silymarin acts directly on cell membranes, it can prevent and cure liver damage.

In the morning, drink a cup of warm/hot water with two table-spoons of fresh squeezed *lemon juice.* The hot water activates the spleen/stomach Meridian which stimulates the movement of blood. The lemon juice detoxifies the liver, astringes the tissues and eliminates the nightly build-up of phlegm.

Charcoal and *chlorophyll,* found in all green plants, are chelators. They bind toxic metals such as lead and mercury to them, pull them out of the liver and flush them out of the body.

Choline, a B vitamin, is essential to healthy liver function. Choline is manufactured in the body by combining folic acid, B_{12} and methionine, an amino acid. Methionine is found in *poultry, nuts, seeds, vegetables* and *fruits.* Choline is also a constituent of lecithin, which can be found in *brewer's yeast, liver* and *wheat germ.*

Linolenic acid, found in *borage oil,* will halt damage to liver cells that have been exposed to toxic substances. *Vitamin E,* as well as *selenium,* also have been shown in research to protect the liver and improve its ability to remove poisons from the system. *Licorice root* is an excellent liver tonic and removes over 1,200 known toxic substances from the body.

The *Reishi mushroom* (Ganoderma) is known as the mushroom of immortality. Reishi is one of the most powerful herbs for enhancing overall liver strength and function as well as the treatment of hepatitis. Japanese doctors use extracts of the Reishi mushroom in the treatment of cancer, especially leukemia and myasthenia gravis. Its polysaccharides are responsible for enhancing immune system function. If you can take herbs or drinks during the body's liver time, II PM to I AM, the liver will be able to extract more energy from them.

To dissipate anger, apply *lavender oil* to a warm cloth like a poultice and place it directly over the liver. Or put a few drops of lavender into a small pot with water, bring it to a soft boil, place a towel over your head and breathe in the steam's aroma to release the anger. The essential oil from *orange* can be used to dissipate internalized anger because it acts as an anti-depressant.

Cancer is a liver issue that needs to be addressed on an individual basis. However, cancer most closely relates to unexpressed anger and creativity, the negative and positive emotional liver expressions. If you or anyone you know contracts cancer, seek immediate medical advice. In addition, you can look at the organ, body part or location of the cancer to determine its emotional root and/or mental causation.

For example, cancer of the bones relates to the kidneys. Look for unresolved emotional or mental issues including unexpressed fears, repressed guilt or shame, stubbornness, rigidity or not being able to listen. The kidneys also rule physical sexual disorders, which includes violations such as incest, molestation and rape. These physical issues have emotional ramifications. Use the emotional and mental harmonizers to start the healing process and to address the cancer on an energetic and attitudinal level. Most important is to work towards the point of forgiveness.

Also, on the physical level, it is imperative to attend to the eliminatory organs. Cleansing the liver, kidneys and colon is mandatory. Also, use herbs, vitamins and minerals to support and enhance the immune system.

The Gall Bladder

The gall bladder is located just under the surface of the liver. It is a green sac that stores the bile produced by the liver. Its main function is to release small quantities of bile into the small intestine to break down fats, proteins and carbohydrates. The gall bladder Meridian, like the bladder Meridian, also covers the body from head to toe.

The gall bladder is considered to be the official in charge of judgments and decisions. The gall bladder is in a central position to receive and release toxins. Thus, it is influential in promoting a state of calm and a sense of well-being. This is important because anger is the most toxic emotion, and excessive and unmanaged anger greatly damages your health and well-being.

Take 1–2 tablespoons of olive oil or flaxseed oil every day to maintain healthy gall bladder function. Flaxseed oil has an expiration date, so make sure it is fresh. Keep it refrigerated and do not heat it. Foods and herbs that strengthen and improve liver function also will have a tonifying effect on the gall bladder.

The liver/gall bladder Meridian's ruling season is the spring, a great time to go on a fast. When the liver/gall bladder Meridians are in balance, the new beginnings you experience will be healthy. Your creativity will blossom, and you will feel enthusiastic about your life. Both Will and Passion are governed by the liver/gall bladder Meridians. When the liver/gall bladder Meridians are healthy, they maintain the balance of your masculine and feminine energies. A healthy liver and gall bladder reflect your ability to plan and carry out your strategies.

To reestablish the flow of energy or clear a physical liver/gall bladder Meridian issue, use conscious breathing to run the color *green* through it. For anger or other liver/gall bladder emotional issues, use the color *turquoise* to access the higher octave of the heart Chakra, the Ananda-Kanta center. For any mental body liver/gall bladder Meridian issues, use the color *gold* to access the mental body element of wisdom.

THE CHAKRA SYSTEMS

The Spiritual discipline of Yoga introduces us to three bodies: physical, astral and causal. Both the emotional and mental bodies are contained within the astral body. The Chakras are subtle energy centers that exist within the Shusumna Nadi—the most important of all Nadis—in the astral body. The Chakras are energy storage depots and have corresponding centers in the spinal cord and nerve plexus in the physical body.

When the Chakra's energy centers are kept clear you will experience Radiant emotional, mental and physical health. On the other hand, repressing emotions, entertaining unhealthy thought forms or engaging in poor eating habits can cause blockages in the Chakras. When the Chakra energy centers are blocked, dis-ease appears in the emotional, mental and physical bodies.

Each of the three Chakra systems found in this section can be used to remove energetic blockages from the astral body. However, because each Chakra system fulfills a specific purpose and raises your frequency to a higher level than the previous system configuration, the three should be applied in the specific order in which they are presented.

Start with the conventional Masculine/Yang Chakra system. This system can be used to clear your Chakras and keep them free of energetic blockages.

Next, use the Feminine/Yin Chakra system configuration and its colors to reestablish the energetic interaction between each Chakra pair, bring your feminine and masculine energies into harmonic balance and open your Spiritual eye.

Finally, use the Divine Child/Integrated Chakra system to bring your vibration into harmonic resonance with the Earth's new and ever increasing frequency.

At the conclusion of each Chakra system, you will find a Chakra Activation Exercise designed to help you dissolve subtle energy blockages, assist healing and also support your quest to achieve Radiant Health.

THE TRADITIONAL/YANG CHAKRA SYSTEM

The energy of the Traditional Chakra system is considered Yang/ Masculine in nature. The configuration of the Yang Chakra system proceeds in a straight line. The line begins at the first Chakra, at the base of the pubic bone, and ascends through each Chakra until it reaches the seventh Chakra, at the crown of the head. The straight line is symbolic of masculine energy.

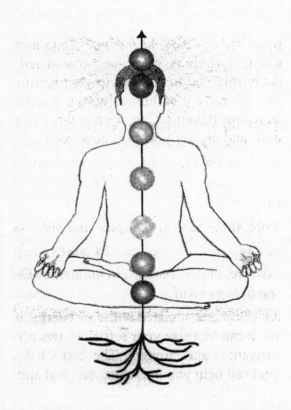

YANG CHAKRA CONFIGURATION

Color chart available at:
www.radiantkeys.com

The Lower Three Chakras, as a group, are considered masculine in nature. The energy of the first three Chakras connects you to Earth as well as to practical issues of living and survival. The first three Chakras are grounding in nature and enable you to access your physical creative energy.

The Fourth Chakra is the heart Chakra and it represents the transition between the upper and lower Chakras. It integrates your masculine and feminine energies. In traditional teachings, meditating on the fourth Chakra opens the heart to love, compassion, empathy and interconnectedness with everything in the world.

The Upper Three Chakras, as a group, are considered feminine in nature. They enable you to connect to your Spiritual nature, the collective consciousness of humanity, the Creator and higher dimensional realms of Spirit. Chakras five through seven are esoteric in nature and enable you to access your Spiritual creative energy.

First Chakra

Chakra location: *At the base of the spine and pubic bone.*
Chakra color: *Red.*   Chakra energy: *Masculine.*
The first Chakra regulates: *Blood, circulation, colon, genitals and the physical body in general.*

The first Chakra is associated with raw energy. Meditation on the first Chakra can increase your self-confidence, courage, will power, assertiveness and strength. The first Chakra's energy is grounding and can help you overcome problems regarding survival and livelihood.

When the first Chakra is open and its energy is cleared, it will dissipate *lethargy, inertia, sluggishness* and *dormancy.* The first Chakra will infuse you with *energy, optimism* and *passion,* enabling you to meet your basic needs such as food and shelter.

Second Chakra

Chakra location: *Just below the navel/belly button.*

Chakra color: *Orange.*   Chakra energy: *Feminine.*

The second Chakra regulates: *Bowels, colon, intestines, prostate and the lower back.*

The second Chakra, being primarily associated with sensual pleasure, is commonly referred to as the sex Chakra. The second Chakra's deeper purpose is to enable you to give and receive the nurturing effects of physical touch such as *hugs, massage* and *being held.* The second Chakra also connects you to your environment by being directly linked to your instinct.

Physical activities—*dance, aerobics, Yoga Asanas* and *making love,* among others—stimulate the second Chakra energy and activate your creative passions.

Lower back pain and its associated problems relate to the emotional need to feel loved and supported. Meditate on the second Chakra to facilitate recovery in areas related to *illness, surgery, addiction, accidents* and *shock.*

Third Chakra

Chakra location: *The solar plexus; just below the point where the ribs meet.*

Chakra color: *Yellow.*   Chakra energy: *Masculine.*

The third Chakra regulates: *Liver, pancreas, central nervous system, skin and endocrine system.*

The third Chakra is known as your center of power. Meditate on the third Chakra to increase your *knowledge of Self;* enhance your *mental clarity, discernment* and *wisdom;* and *empower you to stand for what you believe.* It can also help you recognize, confront, express and release your fear-based beliefs.

Fourth Chakra

Chakra location: *The heart center; middle of the sternum, to the right of the physical heart.*

Chakra color: *Green.*   Chakra energy: *Feminine.*

The fourth Chakra regulates: *Heart and lungs.*

The fourth Chakra governs the *heart* and *relationships*. An open heart Chakra enables you to experience the qualities associated with love's highest Spiritual principle: Agape. It also helps you to embody the qualities of forgiveness, acceptance and compassion. Meditate on the fourth Chakra to experience *joy* and *bliss.*

As the transitional Chakra, the heart marks the starting point on the search between love and truth. The heart enables you to experience the dissolving of separation as it melts the illusion of duality. The heart Chakra also helps you clarify issues of *space, direction, purpose* and *prosperity.*

Fifth Chakra

Chakra location: *The throat.*

Chakra color: *Blue.*   Chakra energy: *Masculine.*

The fifth Chakra regulates: *Colds, coughs, throat issues and the thyroid gland.*

The higher ideals of *truth, loyalty, trust* and *devotion* are governed by the fifth Chakra. A clear and open throat Chakra bridges the distance between the heart and mind, enhancing the skill of discernment and making it possible to allows us to *speak the truth.* Singing also keeps the throat Chakra clear and is a way to communicate your feelings and express love. When the fifth Chakra is open, it magnifies your ability to *communicate clearly, express your ideas with love* and also invokes feelings of *creativity* and *peace,* as well as enhancing your *channeling abilities.*

Sixth Chakra

Chakra location: *The center point between and just above the eyebrows.*
Chakra color: *Indigo.*   Chakra energy: *Feminine.*
The sixth Chakra regulates: *The pineal and pituitary glands, vision, hearing and smell.*

The sixth Chakra is referred to as the Spiritual eye, third eye or Ajna. The Spiritual eye transcends three-dimensional vision and is a doorway to *psychic, clairvoyant, clairsentient* and *clairaudient* experiences. Meditation on the sixth Chakra is best accomplished by closing the eyelids, rolling the eyes upward to the point of the sixth Chakra and breathing fluidly. The sixth Chakra accesses your *intuition, dreams* and *deep memory;* and provides you with *insight* that assists personal transformation. The sixth Chakra can be used to align your personal Will with Divine Will, furthering your awakening to the existence of the Spirit in all things. It also can be used to guide *creative visualizations* and *dissolve stress* and *depression.*

Seventh Chakra

Chakra location: *The crown; the center point of the top of the head.*
Chakra color: *Violet.*   Chakra energy: *Masculine.*
The seventh Chakra regulates: *Life force and all systems in general.*

The seventh Chakra is the direct link to your higher self. Meditation on the seventh Chakra also connects you to Divine source, your guides and angels, other sentient beings and the collective consciousness. The seventh Chakra can help you *transform, purify, heal* and *change* by increasing your conscious and Spiritual awareness. It also can be used to help *alleviate insomnia* and *headaches.*

The Mystery of the Sixth Chakra

There is an interesting anomaly in the traditional Chakra system that merits attention. Each Chakra is imbued with a specific color that emanates from light. However, the sixth Chakra is an exception.

Color arises from one of two sources. The first is light whose spectrum travels from infrared to ultraviolet. The second is pigment colors that are produced by Earth-bound materials not found in the spectrum of light. Examples of pigment colors are black, brown, gray and other earth tones. The anomaly in the traditional Chakra system is that indigo, a color produced by pigment, not light, regulates the sixth Chakra's Spiritual eye.

Consequently, the Spiritual eye, which is responsible for helping you see beyond the illusion of duality and into your Spiritual nature, has been endowed with a pigment color that can actually block your Spiritual vision.

This folly is rooted in the Kali Yuga (see Chapter 1). The world recently passed out of the Dark Ages of the Kali Yuga. It was during the Kali Yuga that the intellectual capacity of humanity was so diminished that human beings worldwide forgot their Divine and Spiritual nature.

The color indigo symbolizes the *"black out"* of Spiritual conscious awareness and humanity's plunge into Spiritual darkness.

Now that the corner has been turned, with every passing year our solar system moves closer and closer to the Grand Center. As more light is infused into the planet, human beings are beginning to regain the memory of their Divine and Spiritual nature and the wisdom that goes along with it. The shift from darkness to light has led to a resurgence in Spiritual growth and reawakening of conscious awareness. The awakening has facilitated the birth, or quite possibly the rediscovery, of the two Chakra systems that resonate at higher vibration levels.

The first, the *Yin Chakra System*, restores balance between the feminine and masculine energies and establishes a color of light at the sixth Chakra to facilitate the opening of the Spiritual eye.

The second, the *Integrated/Divine Child Chakra System*, integrates masculine and feminine energy and raises your frequency, bringing it into harmonic resonance with that of planet Earth.

CHAKRA ACTIVATION EXERCISE I

Sit quietly in a meditative position, back and spine erect, shoes removed, hands in lap and eyes closed. When you feel healthy, use the Yang Chakra system to energize the body. Begin with the first Chakra and follow the system's linear pattern.

Visualize the first Chakra imbued with the color red, spinning in a clockwise direction. If you have trouble visualizing then simply *"feel"* the color red. When you begin to feel a current of energy or a comfortable sensation in the first Chakra move on to the second. Continue visualizing each Chakra in this manner until you complete the pattern and reach the seventh Chakra.

When you experience a specific emotional, mental or physical dis-ease, go to the Index and look up the ailment. Find the Chakra that governs the ailment and use its corresponding colors to clear energy blockages.

To dissolve the energy blockages, visualize the affected Chakra and begin to spin it in a counterclockwise direction. This will begin to dissipate the blocked energy. You might perceive a pigment color such as black, brown or gray being thrown off of the Chakra. This is not unusual. When the pigment color dissolves or the Chakra feels clear, visualize its governing color—for example red at the first Chakra—saturating the Chakra and spin it in a clockwise direction until the color feels bright, energized and lively.

THE YIN CHAKRA SYSTEM

The Yin Chakra system, discovered through a series of in-depth meditations, contains many of the same characteristics as its counterpart, the Yang Chakra system. However, the Yin Chakra system moves you towards the harmonic balance that you need in order to achieve Radiant Health. The Yin system provides you with two significant changes. First, its energetic configuration flows in a circular pattern rather than moving in the straight line found in the Yang system.

Second, although the second and fifth Chakra colors remain the same, the first, third, fourth, sixth and seventh Chakra colors have changed. The change in the color reflects the balance established between the Chakras themselves. Each of the Chakras now resonates with its opposite partner on the color wheel (see page 365). Also, as each color finds its opposite partner, it achieves true resonance to the harmonic number seven, which is considered to be the closest integer to what could be considered a universally complete number.

The Significance of the Yin Chakra Configuration

The Yin Chakra configuration energy begins in the fourth/Heart Chakra and, in a continuous circular spiral, moves down to the third/Solar Plexus Chakra, up to the fifth/Throat Chakra, down to the second/Sex Chakra, up to the sixth/Spiritual Eye Chakra, down to the first/Root Chakra, and finally spirals up and out through the seventh/Crown Chakra.

There are two distinct characteristics in this system that work to restore balance. First, the spiral moves through the Chakras in combinations adding up to the number seven: fourth and third, fifth and second, sixth and first, and seventh by itself.

Second, the Chakra color combinations in the Yin Chakra system, Green and Red, Blue and Orange, Violet and Yellow, are opposite and balancing colors. More about this can be found in the upcoming section, "Colors: Their Meanings and Uses."

Now, take a look at the new interpretations and meanings of the Chakras whose colors have changed from the Traditional Chakra system to the Yin Chakra system.

The First Chakra color changes from Red to Yellow. The issues in the root Chakra shift from survival and work to serving Mother Earth and our fellow human beings. As the root Chakra is opened with the color yellow, it enables you to receive information about how to live in harmony and union with Mother Earth as well as with all other sentient beings.

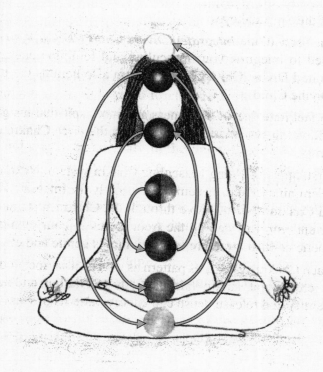

YIN CHAKRA CONFIGURATION

Color chart available at:
www.radiantkeys.com

From the root Chakra, this knowledge can be assimilated. The by-product of putting this information into action is lasting happiness. Corn is a symbolic representation of the root Chakra and its Yellow color. The individual corn kernels are snugly arranged row after row, and interwoven and interconnected with one another in a complete circle. Corn also symbolizes nourishment, the symbolism of unity, interconnectedness and the unending circle of life.

The Third Chakra color changes from Yellow to Red. The third Chakra focus now shifts from self-knowledge, power and mental clarity to intuitive clarity.

Using red to open the third Chakra helps you develop the trust and confidence needed to listen to your intuition. It instills the power to follow your internal messages, even when they do not conform to the protocol of society or to the ideas and beliefs of others. Used in the third Chakra, red can help keep you from engaging in the ego behaviors, or being persuaded by peer pressure to take revenge when you have been hurt, or acting in self-righteous ways that would harm others.

The Fourth Chakra color still contains Green, but now adds Pink as its balancing counterpart. Green now moves to the right/masculine side of the heart Chakra, where it symbolizes the masculine principle of truth. The color pink is brought to the left/feminine side of the heart Chakra where it symbolizes the feminine principle of unconditional love. Together, they create the balance of masculine and feminine energy in your heart and help you to stand for the highest truth: to bring love into your actions.

The fourth Chakra still rules the highest aspect of love, Agape, as well as all relationships. When a question needs to be answered, it is always wise to look into the heart, pray for Divine guidance and then meditate to receive the answer. From the heart, a harmonic answer will always arise.

The Sixth Chakra color changes from Indigo to Violet. The color violet represents the flame of purification. At the sixth Chakra violet burns away the impurities that block the Spiritual eye from being opened. Violet also helps shed light on the illusion of duality and other Mayic manifestations in third-dimensional reality. When the sixth Chakra is opened, the two eyes become one and your Spiritual vision returns. An open third eye helps you recognize and transcend ego behaviors and fearful actions. It also helps to access your heart's love.

The Seventh Chakra color changes from Violet to Clear. Clear stands at the top of the crown, the position of authority. Using the color clear at the seventh Chakra connects you to the entire cosmos and all knowledge. It enables you to dissolve blockages of energy.

As pure light, clear stands on its own. It emits the entire color spectrum from infrared to ultraviolet. Light is absolutely the most powerful color that can be used to assist healing. This is not only because it contains the entire spectrum of color, but because it is the Divine itself.

The amazing healing power of light is just beginning to be understood. Whenever a situation arises in which you experience deep, intense or uncontrollable fear, call on the Divine power of the light: God Itself. Surround yourself with the light and know that you will be fully protected.

Whenever you pray for healing for yourself or others, visualize the purity of light being infused into every part of the individual—entering the opening at the crown Chakra, at the top of the head, and pouring all the way down to the toes. Next visualize the light, starting from the toes, filling the entire body until it reaches the head. As the light reaches the crown Chakra, visualize the crown being closed and see the body radiating in a state of pure light.

THE INTEGRATED/DIVINE CHILD CHAKRA SYSTEM

In the Integrated Chakra system the feminine model provides the creative energy and the masculine energy grounds it. Together they activate The Sacred Trinity of Radiant Health in your subtle energy field to produce the Divine Child.

As your masculine and feminine energies are integrated, a completely new configuration appears. The energy starts from Mother Earth and rises upward through the Yang/masculine linear Chakra pattern. When it reaches the seventh Chakra, instead of launching out into the cosmos, it connects to the Yin/feminine spiral Chakra pattern. The spiral moves in a reverse pattern, circling from the seventh Chakra down to the first. The pattern continues its spiral movement until it reaches the fourth Chakra. The heart is its final resting place. The energies of the Divine Child/Integrated Chakra system enable you to merge with Mother Earth and Father Sky, raising your awareness to a point which enables you to maintain balance with your environment and live in Agape—the highest state of conscious awareness.

These actions can help you create heaven on Earth.

The Integrated/Divine Child Chakra system configuration creates perfect balance by harmonizing the masculine and feminine energy in each Chakra. The Integrated/Divine Child Chakra system transcends dualism by blending Yin and Yang. The Integrated/Divine Child system uses the tertiary colors of light to help you embody your Spiritual life's purpose. The tertiary colors of light are produced by blending the primary colors of light with the secondary colors of light. The Divine Child Chakra system returns you to harmony and union with everything in creation.

In the Integrated/Divine Child Chakra system, every Chakra emits a completely different color than those found in the Yang Chakra system and the Yin Chakra system. As masculine and feminine energy merge to birth the Divine Child, each new Chakra color presents higher vibratory information.

By meditating on each Chakra and using the integrated system's colors, you can raise your frequency and experience a whole new perspective of life. You will see life from the eyes of love. The children now being born on the planet have chosen to experience life from this new perspective as well. They are embodiments of the Integrated/Divine Child Chakra colors. Listed below are the Integrated/Divine Child Chakra system's new colors and their meanings.

Gold is the First Chakra color. Gold represents the wealth of abundance, knowledge and wisdom that is available to you when

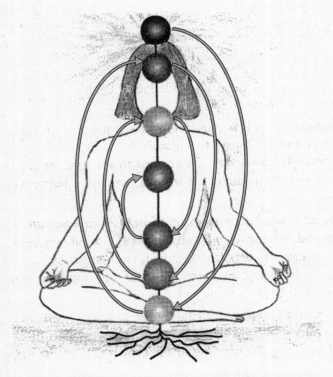

INTEGRATED/DIVINE CHILD CONFIGURATION

Color chart available at:
www.radiantkeys.com

you slow down and honor and respect the natural pace and rhythm of life. Using the color gold to open the first Chakra enhances your ability to live in harmony with Mother Earth, your environment and each other.

Focus on drawing the gold up from Mother Earth's rich veins. Bring the wisdom of the gold into the first Chakra. Gold at the first Chakra reminds you to share the harvests that Earth brings forth, so that the struggle for survival can be released.

Coral is the Second Chakra color. Coral enables you to bring the wisdom of love into your relationships. Coral can help men and women heal the struggles that surround the question of how to express sexual energy in a healthy and non-manipulative way.

Coral balances your sexual energies enabling you to create deeper, more intimate, loving and fulfilling relationships. By using coral to open the second Chakra, you can create the openhearted, nurturing, spontaneous, joyful and happy experiences you want to have with a partner. Coral helps you release the fear, guilt, shame or embarrassment about touching or being touched.

Olive is the Third Chakra color. Olive brings your power center into alignment with feminine leadership qualities. The integrity in power comes from trusting the Creator as well as the goodness in your heart. Opening the third Chakra with olive empowers you to share that love with others. When you embody the feminine quality of trust, you can let go of the ego and fear, and express love. The olive branch stands for peace, and by using olive to open the third Chakra, you can come to know peace.

Magenta is the Fourth Chakra color. Magenta is the highest vibratory color that can be projected into the heart. Magenta can be used to help erase fear from the heart. Magenta enables you to serve humanity with an open heart that is filled with Divine Love. Opening the heart Chakra with magenta enables you to be humble, compassionate and considerate as well as willing to sacrifice your personal desires for the greater good.

Turquoise is the Fifth Chakra color. By using turquoise at the fifth Chakra, the throat can be opened to the most joyous and creative methods of expressing the heart's love to all humanity. Through the throat, the truth can be sung creatively, enthusiastically and with joy. Your communication carries harmonic tones that convey the depth of feelings contained in your heart. By opening the throat Chakra with the color of turquoise, your communication can move into the higher octaves of sound—passing directly from your heart to your throat.

Royal Blue is the Sixth Chakra color. Royal blue can help reveal your illusions. Royal blue can assist you to get a better night's rest and replenishes your vital energy. By using royal blue to open your sixth Chakra, your dreams can help you release subconscious energy. Royal blue enables you connect to higher realms and access your clairvoyance, clairaudience and clairsentience. You can see, hear and feel the guidance that comes from on high. In the awakened state of conscious awareness, the sixth Chakra opens you to experience Divinity. It enables you to release judgments and other ego behaviors that cause you to experience separation.

Deep Magenta is the Seventh Chakra color. Deep magenta enables you to transcend the ego and alleviate its behaviors. The ego will still exist, but you can detach and fully trust that you are under the care, protection and guidance of the Creator. Using deep magenta to open the seventh Chakra enables you to play your part in the Divine play of life. You will be fully aware and not place value on how you are perceived by others as you participate in the play.

CHAKRA ACTIVATION EXERCISE II

1. Close your eyes and roll them upward to the point between the eyebrows and keep your gaze there.

2. Begin with the first Chakra. Touch the physical area of the Chakra and press gently until you feel sensation.

3. Visualize the Chakra spinning counterclockwise.

4. When the Chakra is clear, you may see its color become brighter, or the Chakra energy pulse may feel stronger.

5. When a Chakra feels clear, visualize it spinning clockwise for a few moments.

6. Move to the next Chakra.

7. Be patient as you meditate on the sixth Chakra and in time you will begin to see light or colors, and waves of peace will also descend over you.

NOTE: Any time you clear and balance a specific Chakra, use the opposite Chakra to bring it to the perfect universal balance of the number seven. For example, when you work with the fifth Chakra, include the second Chakra to balance it. The Chakra pairs are: the fourth and third, the fifth and second, the sixth and first. The seventh Chakra stands on its own.

COLORS:
THEIR MEANINGS AND USES

Color plays a major role in your life—from your clothes and jewelry to the car you drive and your home furnishings. Over the ages, color has been used to adjust moods and promote health and well-being. For example, in ancient China, those who suffered epileptic seizures were placed on violet carpets and violet veils were hung over the windows to alleviate their discomfort. Patients with scarlet fever were treated with red lights and dressed in red clothes.

Today, scientific studies are being used to validate the effects color has on health and well-being. For instance, research has found that the color blue is effective in lowering blood pressure and the activity of brain waves, as well as in treating jaundice in newborns. Yellow is a mood elevator, and improves mental clarity and the ability to assimilate information. Pink is used in many prisons because it has demonstrated an ability to neutralize aggressiveness.

The colors you feel drawn to can help you clarify and master emotional, mental or physical challenges, or identify attributes you have or those you aspire to embody. Learning the meanings of color can open you to a deeper and more subtle level of consciousness and increase your self-awareness.

The examination of color presented here is dedicated to colors emitted from the spectrum of light. It contains itemized information that includes the positive supportive attributes along with the challenging attributes associated with each color.

Earth-based pigments such as black, gray, brown and earth tones carry a lower/ego frequency. For example, the characteristics of the popular color black are power, rebellion, independence, silence and individuality. Light, and therefore colors of light, carry a high frequency and can be used to restore balance in the three bodies.

The Color Wheel: Colors of Light

The color wheel contains 12 of the colors emitted by light, which are divided into three subsets: primary, secondary and tertiary. The first three colors discharged by light—*Yellow, Blue* and *Red*—are known as the primary colors. By blending two of the primary colors, three new color combinations, known as the secondary colors, appear:

Red and Blue give birth to *Violet*
Blue and Yellow give birth to *Green*
Yellow and Red give birth to *Orange*

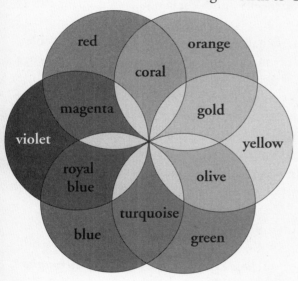

The tertiary colors, the final six colors in the color wheel, arise when the primary colors are combined with the secondary colors.

Orange and Red produce *Coral*
Orange and Yellow produce *Gold*
Yellow and Green produce *Olive*
Green and Blue produce *Turquoise*
Blue and Violet produce *Royal Blue*
Violet and Red produce *Magenta*

Light itself is commonly referred to as the color clear. Although clear does not appear to be a color and is not a visible hue on the color wheel, all colors contained in the color wheel are emitted from it. Because clear quartz crystal contains the entire color spectrum, it is the most powerful conductor of energy.

Two colors of light, pink and deep magenta, do not show up on the color wheel. Pink is produced by shining a light through the color red. Deep magenta is the Yin partner to the Yang color clear. Clear emits all colors of light, and deep magenta absorbs all colors of light. Deep magenta is produced by combining all colors of light. Listed below are key attributes and challenges for each of the 15 colors of light.

Whenever you face a challenge associated with a specific color, use the characteristics of the opposite color to master the challenge and restore balance.

For example, when you are facing challenges represented by the color *blue* such as father issues or depression, use the opposite color, in this case *orange*. Breathe, inhaling the color orange, use it in meditation or wear it. Orange, which represents Assertiveness, Gregariousness, Cheerfulness and Bliss, can help bring the challenge to balance.

The pairs of opposite colors in the color wheel are:

Red–Green	*Yellow–Violet*	*Coral–Turquoise*
Blue–Orange	*Royal Blue–Gold*	*Magenta–Olive*

Color Associations and Their Challenges

Red: Power, Motivation, Grounding, Will, Initiative, Independence, Sexuality, Energy, Authority, Leadership, Optimism, Self-confidence, Determination and Passion.

Challenges: Anger, Resentment, Frustration, Aggression, Impulsiveness, Impatience and Selfishness.

Blue: Peace, Calm, Communication, Loyalty, Trust, Devotion, Patience, Honesty, Sincerity, Reliability, Serenity, Gentleness, Inner Talents and Power.
Challenges: Male models of authority such as Father or the Military, Depression, Apathy, Coldness and Selfish Ambition.

Yellow: Happiness, Knowledge, Brilliance, Enthusiasm, Mental Clarity, Humor, Joy, Assimilation, Illumination, Self-esteem, Discipline and Mastery of Desires.
Challenges: Fear, Criticism, Anxiety, Confusion, Cynicism, Bitterness and Stubbornness.

Violet: Healing, Transformation, Spirituality, Balance of Masculine and Feminine Energy, Intuition, Insight, Change, Service, Meditation, Relaxation, Contemplation, Majesty, Purification and Royalty.
Challenges: Escapism, Grief, Intolerance, Injustice, Hidden Anger, Arrogance and Martyrdom.

Green: Growth, Space, Decisions, Money, Harmony, Balance, Integrity, Direction, Health, Seeker of Truth, Heart, Fertility, Nurturing, Generosity, Acceptance, Discernment and Compromise.
Challenges: Decision-making, Jealousy, Envy, Being Cramped, Pessimism, Rigidity, Vindictiveness and Emotional Repression.

Orange: Bliss, Gregariousness, Pleasure, Rapture, Aspiration, Renunciation, Freedom, Gut Feelings, Cheerfulness, Sociability, Assertiveness, Organization and Discipline.
Challenges: Shock, Trauma, Co-dependence, Dependency, Confusion, Intolerance, Possessiveness, Overindulgence and Lust.

Coral: Wisdom to Love Ourselves, Good Fortune, Higher Intuition, Spontaneity, Joy in Love, Happiness and Self-analysis.
Challenges: Unrequited Love, Undeclared or Hidden Love, Aloneness, Isolation and Resolving Frustrations.

Gold: Wisdom, Deep Self Value, Exaltation, Deep Joy, Beauty, Abundance, Wealth, Justice, Enlightenment and Holiness.
Challenges: Irrational Fears, Self-doubt, Phobias, Control, Nervousness, Greed and Deep Confusion.

Olive: Feminine Qualities of Leadership, Peace, Transmutation and Completion.
Challenges: Leadership, Joy, Bitterness, Envy, Inner Awareness, Power Issues and Control.

Turquoise: Creativity, Communication from One to Many, Creative Expression, Humanitarian, Social Consciousness, Idealism, Independence and Artistry.
Challenges: Expressing Feelings, Suppression, Sadness, Awareness and Foolishness.

Royal Blue: Mysticism, Clairvoyance, Clairaudience, Clairsentience, Objectivity and Reverence.
Challenges: Aloofness, Rigidity, Isolation, Resistance and Loneliness.

Magenta: Divine Love, Compassion, Cooperation, Loving Attention to Detail and Caring in All Matters.
Challenges: Searching for Divine Love Outside of the Human Experience.

Clear: Integration, Clarity, Purity, Understanding of Suffering, Truth, Honesty, Deep Reflection, Simplicity, Determination and Being an Empty Vessel.
Challenges: Not Seeing Clearly, Washed Out, Unshed Tears, Suffering and Detoxification.

Pink: Unconditional Love and the Ability to Give and Receive.
Challenges: Not Being Able to Receive Love.

Deep Magenta: The Perfect Love of the Mother.
Challenges: Deep magenta is the only color in the spectrum of light that has no associated challenges.

Using Color to Restore Balance in the Chakras

By using conscious breathing to infuse a specific color into a Chakra on the in-breath and to release the energy blockages on the exhale, balance in the Chakra can be restored. If a color is difficult to visualize during meditation, then just think about it or feel it. The healing vibrations and characteristics of the color will be picked up and drawn to the place where it is being directed by the breath.

IMMUNE-BOOSTING NUTRIENTS

Excess stress and tension, air and water pollution and mineral-depleted soil can lead to a weakened immune system. To replace the nutrients lost due to personal and environmental factors, add vitamins and minerals to your daily nourishment regimen. When used as an adjunct to meals in the dosages shown, these nine vitamins and minerals can improve overall immune system function.

Vitamin C. 1000 mg: Protects against viral infection by strengthening connective tissue and neutralizing toxic substances released by phagocytes. Vitamin C contains antiviral, antibacterial and anticancer properties. Five hundred milligrams of vitamin C per day increases levels of glutathione by 50%.

Vitamin A. 5,000 IU: Normalizes cell division and helps mucus membranes maintain their structural integrity to keep invaders out. Deficiency causes thymus shrinkage (impairing the immune system), susceptibility to infections, colds, flu and increased time for healing of wounds, including stomach ulcers.

Vitamin E. 400–800 IU: Used in conjunction with selenium and vitamin C, vitamin E is a potent immune protector. Vitamin E increases resistance to infection, cell-mediated immunity and phagocytosis. An active antioxidant, vitamin E reduces damage caused by stress. Vitamin E also is beneficial for cardiovascular disease, diabetes, cancer, skin disorders, arthritis, PMS and inflammation.

Zinc. **25 mg:** The most important mineral to the thymus gland. Required for cell-mediated immunity and proper cell division and DNA synthesis. Zinc increases interleukin-2, which authorizes cytotoxic T-cells to attack invaders. Zinc increases thymulin and reduces excess copper in the body's tissues which is a leading cause of chronic fatigue syndrome.

Selenium. **100 mcg:** A potent free radical scavenger, selenium enables the immune system to mobilize T-cells and natural killer cells to destroy pathogenic bacteria and viruses. Deficiency causes poor resistance to viruses and bacteria, reduces T-cell activity and antibody production. Selenium use increases interluekin-2, important in activating natural killer cell activity. One or two fresh Brazil nuts provide an adequate amount of selenium to the daily diet.

Coenzyme Q10. **30 mg:** A precursor to enzyme function, coenzyme Q10 increases antibody production and macrophage activity. After age 50, Coenzyme Q10 levels have been shown to drop by 50% of what they were at age 20. Coenzyme Q10 has antiviral, antibacterial and antitumor effects.

Reduced L-glutathione. **75 mg–150 mg:** This amino acid is important in DNA synthesis and repair, protein synthesis, amino acid transport and detoxification of toxins and carcinogens. Reduced L-glutathione enhances the immune system and provides protection from oxidation. Environmental allergic reaction can be alleviated with 200-500 mg of L-glutathione taken daily. Reduced L-glutathione enhances cellular oxygenation.

Vitamin B-6 (**in a B complex**). **50 mg:** Inadequate levels of B-6 causes the thymus to shrink and reduces the amount of available thymulin. T-cell activity diminishes as do B-cells and antibodies. Interleukin-2 is also reduced, disabling the natural killer cells, which in turn raises the risk of infection and compromises the immune system.

Magnesium. **100 mg:** Responsible for more than 300 enzymatic reactions in the body. Magnesium deficiency causes an increase in pro-inflammatory conditions, as well as excesses in the production of the free radicals seen in chronic fatigue syndrome, fibromyalgia and rheumatoid conditions.

TONIC HERBALISM

The ancient Chinese art of tonic herbalism was recently introduced to the West. The tonics comprise a special classification within the Chinese herbal pharmacopoeia. Of its over 6,000 herbs, the tonics comprise only 60 herbs or approximately 1% of the entire pharmacopoeia. Shen Nong, the father of Chinese herbalism, created a system that placed every herb into one of three classifications: *Inferior, General or Superior.*

Tonics are categorized as superior herbs. Tonic herbs have no medicinal value and are not used to treat or prevent illness. Instead, they are traditionally used to enhance one's vital life force energy, restore and support the immune system and increase longevity. Taken regularly, the tonic effect of superior herbs accrues over time, providing cumulative benefits. The adaptive energy contained in tonic herbs decreases stress and tension; enhances the flow of subtle energy through the Nadis, Meridians and Chakras; and awakens you to your Spiritual nature enabling you to enjoy Radiant Health.

The Chinese system of herbal classification is more than 5,000 years old. Before an herb was bestowed with the lofty status of being a tonic or superior herb, it was subjected to exhaustive study. The empirical research methods used to ascertain its qualities and actions lasted not only for months or years, but for centuries. To be classified as a tonic, an herb had to comply with the first law of Chinese herbalism: do no harm. Over the course of centuries it had to meet six rigorous qualifications. They are:

1. *The herb has to possess profound health-promoting actions.*

2. *The herb must be shown as an aid in increasing longevity.*

3. *The herb must improve one's overall emotional and Spiritual well-being, which produces happiness.*

4. *Used consistently and in moderation over a long period of time, the herb has to be found to have no negative side effects.*

5. *The herb must be easy to digest and must taste good.*

6. *One of the "Three Treasures" must be contained in the herb in such abundant proportions that it can strengthen that Treasure in everyone who consumes it.*

Taoist sages believed that every human being was composed of Three Treasures: Jing, Chi and Shen, described below. Every herb classified as a tonic has to contain, support and accentuate one or more of the Three Treasures.

The Three Treasures

Jing, the first treasure, describes your essence, life force or primal energy. Jing is a combination of Yin and Yang energy. Every individual is born with a finite amount of Jing, which is predetermined by your ancestral heritage and genetic make-up. The quantity of Jing determines the length and vitality of your life, and can be influenced by engaging in Spiritual practices and living a balanced lifestyle.

Jing is akin to the wax of a candle: when a candle's wax burns away, its flame of life is extinguished. Traditional Chinese medicine asserts that Jing is contained in the kidneys with its greatest concentrations being contained in the adrenals and reproductive system. Jing is depleted by acute or chronic stress, and/or overindulgence, excess or extremes in sex, emotions, work, poor diet and childbirth. *Jing tonics* such as *Ho sho wu, Cordyceps, Reishi, Schizandra, Rehmannia, Morinda, Epimedium, Lycium fruit, Cistanche, Polygonatum sibericum* and *Eucommia* help reduce the depletion of your life force energy and replenish and rebuild your deep reserves.

Chi, the second treasure, fortifies your energy and blood and is produced by extracting prana—life force energy—from the air you breathe and the food you eat. Chi helps you to adapt to your environment and function effectively within it. When you are faced with stressful situations and have ample amounts of chi, you handle them with a clear mind and a calm heart. *Chi tonics* such as *Codonopsis, Atractylodes* and *Ginseng* are said to strengthen digestive assimilation and the functions of the respiratory system. *Ligusticum* and *Tang Kuei* build blood. *Astragulus* and *Reishi* are believed to contain potent immune system modulating activity.

Shen is the third and most important treasure of all. Shen refers to that Spirit that resides in your heart. It is expressed as compassion, generosity, kindness, acceptance, love, patience, peace, forgiveness and tolerance. Shen is the quality that allows you to rise above ego pettiness, transcending duality to see all sides of an issue and embracing the wisdom in the oneness of all things. Shen tonics such as *Reishi, Polygala, Spirit poria, Albizzia, Asparagus root* and *Zizyphus* keep you firmly grounded in the present moment, fully aware of all that takes place in your environment and your inner self.

The "Cream of the Crop" of Tonic Herbs

Listed below are four *"Cream of the crop"* tonic herbs. Each is outstanding and powerful in its application and can be used with regularity. Before taking any herbs, check with your healthcare professional.

Ganoderma (**Reishi mushroom**). Known as "The Mushroom of Immortality," for thousands of years this has been the prized tonic herb in the Chinese pharmacopoeia. In research it has been shown to strengthen the immune system specifically by boosting the immunoglobulins, leukocytes and T-cells. It has a tonifying effect on the liver, helping to regulate its function and regenerate liver cells. It is also a powerful antioxidant.

Astragulus. Another very powerful herb in the Chinese tonic pharmacopoeia, Astragulus contains immune modulating and stimulating properties. In China, the combination of Astragulus and Reishi has long been known as *"The Great Protector"* because each has such powerful immune modulating factors. Traditionally, it has been used to improve metabolic function and strengthen muscles, but it is also known for its powerful properties as an antioxidant. Astragulus contains many trace minerals and micro-nutrients, and it increases wei-chi, or a person's own protective energy. Astragulus also strengthens the lungs and it has been shown to diminish the effects of chemotherapy.[1]

Ginseng. One of the most popular and widely used tonics in the world, Ginseng helps the spleen and lungs extract energy from the food you eat and air you breathe. Ginseng is an adaptogen that contains saponins called ginsenosides, a substance that helps the body achieve and maintain homeostasis and restore energy.

Ginseng produces an abundance of energy with no side effects when used in moderation. Because it regenerates energy, quality Ginseng will actually help you sleep if you need rest. When harvested before maturity, Ginseng can cause restlessness. Mature roots are at least six years old, and roots twenty years or older are preferred because, it is said, greater Spirit and wisdom energy are contained in their roots. Wild or semi-wild roots are preferred to commercially cultivated roots because they are said to contain more Spirit energy.

Schizandra. A renowned beauty tonic that preserves youth, makes the skin soft, moist and radiant, Schizandra has been consumed by Chinese royalty. Schizandra is one of a very few tonics that contains all three treasures. Also, it is said to enter all twelve Meridians. Schizandra is considered to be a powerful tonic for the brain and memory, improves sexual stamina and function, and strengthens the entire body.

GEMS AND CRYSTALS

When a blockage exists in the subtle energy bodies, gems and crystals can be used to restore their free flow of energy. Gems and crystals provide you with an opportunity to dissolve the blockage and affect healing by harmonizing and balancing the emotional, mental and physical bodies.

Resonance is the principle power behind the ability of gems and crystals to affect healing. As you know, the cellular structure of the human body is electro-magnetic in nature and resonates at 7.8 Hertz. Gems and crystals are also electro-magnetic in nature and resonate at a higher frequency. When a crystal is placed on or in proximity to your body, the rate at which your cells vibrate will attempt to match the higher vibration rate of the crystals.

When you place gems or crystals on a dis-eased body area, Meridian or Chakra, you can meditate and attune yourself to the crystal's resonance. The crystals and gems listed in the Meridian charts can be used to assist in dissolving the specific physical, mental and emotional blockages of energy.

Also, it is important to keep the vibrational energy of your gems and crystals clean and clear. *A gem or crystal will lose its luster when it needs to be cleared of lower vibrations.* After working with your gems and crystals, place them in a bowl of dry sea salt to replenish their energy. A few hours up to one day is usually all it takes to restore their sheen. When their sparkle returns, the energy in your gems and crystals has been rejuvenated. Sea salt clears negative energy from crystals or you can wash them in cold water to revitalize them.

To infuse more Yang/active energy into your crystals, place them out in the sun. To imbue more Yin/receptive energy, place your crystals out under a full moon. For more grounded energy, place your crystals in the Earth for a day or two. For example, hematite is an excellent stone for grounding, but to ground yourself in love, put a rose quartz in the Earth for a day or two. When you remove the rose quartz from the Earth, its grounding energy will enable you to focus more energy on expressing love.

Crystal and Gem Meditation

To assist your healing process, restore the free flow of energy to the subtle energy bodies, and free blocked energy from the emotional, mental or physical bodies, follow the steps below:

1. *When You Experience a Dis-ease:* choose the appropriate crystal or gem from the Meridian that regulates the emotional, mental or physical dis-ease. For example, choose one or more variety of stones from the Lung and Large Intestine Meridian to use for asthma.

2. *Place the Stones in Your Left and Right Hand.* The left side of the body receives energy. The right side of the body sends energy. Or, you can place the crystals on the body at the point of discomfort, on the affected Meridian, Chakra or wherever you feel drawn to place them.

3. *Prepare to Meditate.* Remove your shoes, sit or lie down. Close your eyes and keep your spine straight. Get as comfortable as possible and begin to practice conscious breathing.

4. *Set an Intention to Absorb the Healing Vibrations of the Crystals.* Your intention will enable you to commune with the crystals, raising your own vibration to that of the crystals and making it far more likely that your energy blockages can be dissolved.

5. *Place Your Attention on the Stones and Begin to Meditate.* Take a few moments to quiet the mind. Begin to focus on conscious breathing and then direct your attention to the stones.

6. *When You Inhale,* feel and visualize the energy from the stone in your left hand entering the left side of your body, and then passing into the right side of your body.

7. *When You Exhale,* visualize the energy flowing out of the right side of the body. Allow the energy to pass through the stone in

your right hand. As it completely exits the body, see Mother Earth absorbing the energy.

8. *Continue This Circular Motion Meditation.* On the next inhale, feel and visualize Mother Earth sending new energy into the stone in your left hand. Continue to inhale and exhale using this circular motion meditation. When you feel completely calm and at peace, the meditation is complete.

9. *Clear Your Crystals When You Have Completed the Meditation.* After working with your gems and crystals, place them in a bowl of sea salt, water or earth to replenish their energy. When the crystal's sparkle returns, its energy has been rejuvenated.

SIX EXERCISES TO ASSIST THE HEALING PROCESS

When an emotional, mental or physical dis-ease arises, the following exercises can be used in conjunction with the information provided in the Meridian, Chakra and Color sections to assist the healing process. Or, the information can be used to keep the subtle energy systems flowing freely, the three bodies healthy and vital, and yourself firmly on the path of Radiant Health. Also, you can establish a set time every day to check in with your Spirit Child to see if there is something subtle to work on, or a minor problem that slipped by you during the course of the day.

1. *Create and Use Affirmations and Mantras.*

When you uncover a dis-ease-producing emotional or mental pattern, use the emotional and mental harmonizer lists in the Meridian charts to create affirmations. Recite the affirmations as incantations.

Keep your affirmations simple and write them out. Keep repeating them in your thoughts, and speak them with Passion. Make a commitment to practice them several times throughout the day. For example, if you are constantly angry, look up anger in the Index. You will find that anger can be traced to the liver–gall bladder Meridian. Use the emotional and mental harmonizers and your affirmations might sound like this:

A) *My creative energy is flowing freely.*

B) *I transform my anger into motivation.*

C) *I feel confident and prepared.*

2. *Reestablish the Meridian's Subtle Energy Flow.*

Meditate on the blocked Meridian. Visualize energy flowing uninterrupted through the affected Meridian and also through its partner. It might be helpful the first time you do this to trace the path with the index finger while you refer to the appropriate Meridian diagram.

For example, start at the base of the big toenail and visualize energy flowing through the external liver Meridian pathway. Next, connect the last point of the external liver Meridian—the intercostal space between the sixth and seventh ribs—to the first point of the internal liver Meridian pathway.

Do the same with the gall bladder Meridian. Start at the first gall bladder point, one-half finger width behind the outer corner of the eye. Visualize the energy flowing freely until it reaches the last point of the external gall bladder Meridian, at the outside corner of the base of the fourth toenail. Continue on and connect it to the first point of the internal gall bladder Meridian pathway.

Continue until you feel the energy flowing in a smooth cycle through both Meridians.

3. *Bring One of the Meridian's Specific Colors into Your Meditation.*

For example, visualize the color *green* flowing through the *liver Meridian* when a physical liver discord exists. When a gall bladder discord exists, visualize the color *olive* flowing through the *gall bladder Meridian.*

Visualize the color *gold* flowing through both Meridians when a *mental body liver–gall bladder* discord exists.

When an *emotional body liver–gall bladder* discord exists, visualize the color *turquoise* flowing through both Meridians.

4. *Clear the Energy Blockages from the Chakras.*

Meditate on the affected Chakras to clear blockages and restore the free flow of energy. Use the colors from the traditional Chakra system to assist the emotional, mental or physical dis-ease clearing process.

For example, if the dis-ease affects the lower back, use the second Chakra and its traditional Chakra color—orange—to assist the healing process. If the dis-ease pertains to the lungs, use the fourth Chakra and its traditional Chakra color—green.

Visualize the Chakra revolving in a counterclockwise direction from left to right on the body. As it spins, visualize the blocked energy being hurled off of the Chakra. The unhealthy energy might appear dull, discolored or another color such as black, brown or gray.

When the Chakra feels clear, its color becomes lustrous and radiant, or you feel a physical sensation of comfort in the Chakra area, begin to rotate the Chakra in a clockwise direction, from right to left on the body.

5. *Visualize the Affected Physical Area Being Healed.*

When the dis-ease affects the physical body, meditate on the area of the dis-ease. Visualize the affected area being healed and the body being restored to a state of health and vitality.

Spend ten minutes in the morning, afternoon and evening visualizing the area and the entire body being healthy. When possible, practice the visualization during the affected body part's Meridian peak time. For example, for a broken bone, try to meditate during the kidney Meridian's peak time: 5 to 7 PM.

Use the associated Meridian's color for physical healing in your meditation. For example, if the physical dis-ease is a broken bone, then use the kidney Meridian's physical body associated color—red—in your meditation to help facilitate healing.

6. *Strengthen Your Vital Energy by Following These Routines Every Day:*

   1. *Drink teas made from tonic herbs.*

   2. *Wear Meridian and Chakra colors,* and *gems and crystals* that relate to your emotional, mental or physical body areas that need to be strengthened.

   3. *Massage the Meridians,* and any other related areas that are associated with pain or tension, or that relate to an emotional, mental or physical issue.

   4. *Meditate regularly on the Meridians and Chakras* to keep their energy clear, free-flowing and fluid.

Notes

CHAPTER 1. STARTING THE JOURNEY

1. Adapted from *The Holy Science*—Swami Sri Yukteswar, Self-Realization Fellowship, 1990.

CHAPTER 2. THE WORLD'S JOURNEY TO RADIANT HEALTH

1. Adapted from *The Late Great Planet Earth*—Hal Lindsey.

2. Hopi prophecies are etched in stone at Oraibi.

3. Lecture by Professor Lani Guanier—March 2000, Pacifica Radio—KPFK.

4. Prophecies are summarized and adapted from *The Hopi Survival Kit*—Tomas E. Mails.

5. Lakota prophecies are handed down by oral tradition.

6. Adapted from *The Delphi Associate*, Vol. 2, Issue #13, 1994—Sean David Morton, Publisher/Editor.

7. According to Frank Water—*Mexico Mystique*.

CHAPTER 6. CHOOSING THE PROPER BREATHING METHOD

1. Commenting on the incorruptible state of the physical body after the master Paramahansa Yogananda passed into Mahasamadi, "The absence of any signs of visual decay in the body of Paramahansa Yogananda offers the most extraordinary case in our experience. No visible disintegration was visible in his body, even twenty days after death. No indication of mold was visible on his skin, and no visible desiccation took place in the bodily tissues. No odor of decay took place at any time. This state of perfect preservation of a body is, so far as we know from mortuary annals, an unparalleled one."

2. *Breathe! You Are Alive*—Thich Nhat Hanh, Parallax Press, 1996.

CHAPTER 8.   THE SACRED TRINITY OF RADIANT HEALTH

    1. When God Was a Woman—Merlin Stone, Harcourt Brace, 1976.

CHAPTER 13.   SADNESS: THE FEMININE EMOTION

    1. Martin Practel—Lecture on Grief and Praise, Cassette Tape.

CHAPTER 14.   LAUGHTER: THE EMOTION OF THE DIVINE CHILD

    1. The sedimentation rate is derived from a diagnostic test that measures the speed with which red blood cells settle in a test tube—a normal illness might produce a reading of 30 or even 40; however when the rate is measured beyond 60 or 70 it indicates a more serious illness.

CHAPTER 19.   THE EMOTIONAL BODY CENTER: LOVE AND AGAPE

    1. Adapted from *Vision of Sai Book* 2—Reta Bruce, Weiser Publications, 1996.

    2. From a brochure introducing the Dalai Lama's teaching retreat in Los Angeles, California, May 2000.

CHAPTER 21.   THOUGHT FORMS

    1. Adapted from *The Divine Romance*—Paramahansa Yogananda, Self-Realization Publications, 1986.

CHAPTER 23.   THE POWER OF WILL

    1. Adapted from *The Divine Romance*—Paramahansa Yogananda, Self-Realization Publications, 1986.

    2. The portion of the brain stem between the spinal cord and the pons that is also known as the Mouth of God. *The Divine Romance*—Paramahansa Yogananda, Self-Realization Publications, 1986.

    3. Adapted from *The Divine Romance*—Paramahansa Yogananda, Self-Realization Publications, 1986.

CHAPTER 25.   FEAR

    1. A commencement speech given by Winston Churchill at Oxford University shortly after World War II, circa 1945.

    2. *The Bhagavad Gita on Tape*—Jacob Needleman, narrator, 1987.

CHAPTER 27. THE EGO'S COMPONENTS OF SEPARATION

1. *Global Spin*—Susan Beder, Chelsea Green Publishing, 1997.
2. *Global Spin*—Susan Beder, Chelsea Green Publishing, 1997.
3. *The Wall Street Journal*, Op-ed article written by Dennis T. Avery, April 1, 1993.

CHAPTER 31. THE OUTER LAYER OF THE PHYSICAL BODY

1. *"Feeding Frenzy,"* *Newsweek*, May 27, 1991. Charles B. Simone, M.D., Cancer and Nutrition, McGraw-Hill.
2. Surgeon General C. Everett Koop—Exact date unknown.
3. *Cancer: Causes, Prevention and Treatment*—Paavo Airola, Ph.D., N.D., Health Plus, Phoenix AZ, 1974.
4. *Cancer: Causes, Prevention and Treatment*—Paavo Airola, Ph.D., N.D., Health Plus, Phoenix AZ, 1974.
5. *The Master Cleanser*—Stanley Burroughs, Burroughs Books, Reno NV, 1993.

CHAPTER 32. THE SECOND LAYER: THE PHYSICAL BODY'S SUBTLE ENERGY SYSTEMS

1. *A Cancer Therapy*—Max Gerson, M.D., The Gerson Institute, 1958.
2. *Hoxsey: The Quack Who Cured Cancer?*—American Media.
3. *The Conquest of Cancer: Vaccines and Diet*—Virginia Livingston-Wheeler and Edmond G. Addeo, New York, 1984.
4. *How You Can Beat the Killer Diseases*—Harold Harper and Michael L. Culbert, Arlington House, 1977.
5. *A Cancer Therapy*—Max Gerson, M.D., The Gerson Institute 1958.
6. Note 6, page 292, needs reference

CHAPTER 33. THE PHYSICAL BODY CENTER: ACTION AND SERVICE

1. From the *How to Live* series entitled *Healing by God's Unlimited Power*. Paramahansa Yogananda, Self-Realization Publications, 1985.

CHAPTER 34. AWAKENING: THE JOURNEY TO LIGHT

1. Front page article in *The Los Angeles Times,* Sept. 4, 1998.

2. 1998 study by John Astin, Ph.D., Stanford University. David Eisenberg, M.D., and colleagues, Harvard Medical School, *Nutrition in Complementary Care*—Fall 1998, Vol. 1 Number 1.

Bibliography

Anatomy of an Illness—Norman Cousins, Bantam Books, 1979.

An Outline of Chinese Acupuncture—The Academy of Traditional Chinese Medicine, Foreign Language Press—Reprinted in USA.

Awakening to Zero Point: The Collective Initiation—Greg Braden, Radio Publications, 1993.

Aura-Soma—Irene Dalichow and Mike Booth, Hay House, 1996.

Breathe! You Are Alive—Thich Nhat Hanh, Parallax Press, 1996.

Chinese Tonic Herbalism—Ron Teegarden, Japan Publications.

Crystal Enlightenment—Katrina Raphaell, Aurora Press, 1985.

The Crystal Kingdom—Melody, Earth-Love Publishing, 1999.

The Divine Romance—Paramahansa Yogananda, Self-Realization Fellowship, 1986.

Essentials of Chinese Acupuncture—Foreign Language Press, Beijing, China.

Global Spin—Sharon Beder, Chelsea Green Publishing, 1997

Heal Your Body—Louise Hay, Hay House, 1988.

The Holy Science—Swami Sri Yukteswar, Self-Realization Fellowship, 1990.

The Hopi Survival Kit—Thomas E. Mails, Penguin Books, 1997.

Hoxsey: The Quack Who Cured Cancer?—American Media Video.

Human Anatomy—Van De Graaff, McGraw-Hill Publishing, 1998.

The Immune System Cure—Lorna R. Vanderhaeghe and Patrick J.D. Bouic, Ph.D., Prentice Hall, 1999.

Intermediate & Advanced Acupressure Course Booklet—Michael Reed Gach, Acupressure Institute, 1984.

The Last Hours of Ancient Sunlight—Thom Hartmann, Harmony Books, 1998.

The Late Great Planet Earth—Hal Lindsey, Zondervon Publishing House, 1977.

The Legend of King Asoka—John S. Strong, Motilal Banarsidass, 1989.

Lightshift 2000—Ken Kalb, Lucky Star Press, 1998.

Man's Eternal Quest—Paramahansa Yogananda, Self-Realization Fellowship, 1986.

The Master Cleanser—Stanley Burroughs, Burroughs Books, Reno NV, 1993.

The Mayan Factor—Jose Arguelles, Bear & Co. Publications, 1987.

The Miracle of Color—Vicki Wall, Hay House.

Mysterious Places—Jennifer Westwood, Barnes and Noble, 1997.

The Prophet—Kahlil Gibran, Alfred A. Knopf Inc., New York, 1979.

The Sivananda Companion to Yoga—The Sivananda Yoga Center, 1983.

Smart Medicine for a Healthier Child—Janet Zand, Rachel Walton, Bob Roundtree, Avery Publishing, 1994.

Staying Healthy with the Seasons—Elson Haas, Celestial Arts, 1981.

Thought Forms—Annie Besant and C.W. Leadbeater, Quest Publications, 1969.

Toxic Deception—Dan Fagin, Marianne Lavelle and The Center for Public Integrity, Common Courage Press, 1999.

Understanding Nutrition—Witney, Rolfes, West Publishing, 1996.

Vision of Sai Book 1—Reta Bruce, Weiser Publications, 1996.

Vision of Sai Book 2—Reta Bruce, Weiser Publications, 1996.

What the Buddha Taught—Haw Trai Foundation Press, no date.

Wheels of Life—Anodea Judith, Ph.D., Llewellyn Publishing, 1987.

When God Was a Woman—Merlin Stone, Harcourt Brace, 1976.

Index